Quality Assurance and Quality Management in Pharmaceutical Industry

Quality Assurance and Quality Management in Pharmaceutical Industry

Prof. Y. Anjaneyulu

Director
Institute of Science and Technology
Jawaharlal Nehru Technological University
Kukatpally, Hyderabad-500 072.

Dr. R. Marayya

Consultant to Pharmaceutical Industries
Mehdipatnam, Hyderabad-500 028.

Pharma Med PRESS An Imprint of Pharma Book Syndicate

PharmaMed Press
An imprint of Pharma Book Syndicate

A unit of BSP Books Pvt. Ltd.

4-4-316, Giriraj Lane,
Sultan Bazar, Hyderabad - 500 095.

Published by :

PharmaMed Press

An imprint of Pharma Book Syndicate

A unit of BSP Books Pvt. Ltd.

4-4-316, Giriraj Lane, Sultan Bazar, Hyderabad - 500 095.
Phone: 040-23445605, 23445688; Fax: 91+40-23445611
E-mail: info@pharmamedpress.com

ISBN : 978-93-52300-73-0 (HB)

JAWAHARLAL NEHRU TECHNOLOGICAL UNIVERSITY

Dr. K. RAJAGOPAL
VICE-CHANCELLOR

Kukatpally,
Hyderabad - 500 072
Andhra Pradesh (India).
Grams : "Technology"
Phone. 040 - 23156109 (O)
Fax : 040 - 23156112
E-mail: vcjntu@jntuap.ac.in
www.jntu.ac.in

Foreword

The extent and implementation of Quality Assurance (QA) and Quality Management Systems (QMS) in Pharmaceutical Industry is a measure of the degree of scientific, technical and managerial skills adopted by it in the manufacturing process. In the present global competition the total quality management with appropriate QA & QM synthesis is considered as an integral part of business management and to meet the corresponding skilled manpower requirements, education and advanced training in this specialized field is highly essential.

In this context this book written by Prof. Y. Anjaneyulu with his rich teaching and R & D experience and his student Dr. R. Marayya with his industrial experience as consultant covering all latest concepts on QA and QMS with good practical examples, will be useful for graduates and postgraduates of pharmacy, chemistry and practicing professionals in this field.

The QA & QMS concepts being very recent origin in the Indian context very few books are available and I congratulate the authors for bringing out this book at a right time on a very important specialised field of great industrial relevance.

K. Rajagopal

Prologue

In recent times, advanced drug design, production processes and sophisticated analytical instrumentation have added new dimensions to the complexity of industrial pharmaceutical production process leading to the necessity of extensive and indepth implementation of Quality Assurance (QA) and Quality Management Systems (QMS). Further, new regulations and legislations concerning product quality requirements in pharmaceutical industry and proactive role played by regulatory agencies by way of enforcing legal penalties for non conformity of quality standards have increased the responsibility of the manufacturer for the rigorous quality control of the product. In view of this, implementation of the Quality Assurance and Quality Management System concepts are playing a vital role in the production and global marketing in pharmaceutical industry.

Thus, understanding of basic concepts and recent developments in QA and QMS has become very important both for scientific and management personnel and graduate and post-graduate students of Pharmacy, Industrial and Analytical Chemistry, chemical technology and other related disciplines who are likely to serve the manpower requirements of various pharmaceutical industries.

This book authored by Prof. Y. Anjaneyulu, Director, IST, JNT University, Hyderabad, very senior Professor and reputed R & D Scientist and Dr. R. Marayya, a well-known pharma consultant gives the overall view of QA and QMS with reference to pharmaceutical industry. QMS, GLP, GMP, Statistical methods in quality control and quality audit are discussed very lucidly and with latest information and guidelines. The information presented in Chapter 4 on Methods of Analytical Quality Assurance is very useful as it provides many possible solutions for routine practice.

In appendix, the latest information on the International Standards on QMS, GLP and GMP for pharmaceutical industry are included which will be useful as a ready reference.

As very few books are available on this important subject, this book will be very useful as text book for students of both graduate and post-graduate classes in Pharmacy, Analytical Chemistry and allied subjects. It shall serve as ready reference for scientific and management personnel working in various pharmaceutical industries for understanding the basic concepts and implementation of QA and QMS with latest guidelines.

I am happy to write the Prologue for this book and congratulate Prof. Y. Anjaneyulu and his student Dr. R. Marayya for bringing out a text book on this very important topic of great relevance in pharmaceutical field.

Prof. (Dr.) Chandrakant Kokate

Former Vice-Chancellor, Kakatiya University,
Former President, Pharmacy Council of India,
Former E.C. Member & Chairman.
All India Board of Pharmacy, A.I.C.T.E.

Sri Venkateshwara Vaibhav Apartments,
H.No. 3-3-935, Flat No. 102,
Kutbhiguda, Kachiguda, Hyderabad-27

Preface

Quality Assurance (QA) is a measure of the degree of sophistication of managerial, scenititic and technical tools used in the design and development and implementation of production process of any industry. QA is the most vital function of Total Quality Management in pharmaceutical industry and is considered as an integral part of business and market. To meet the internationally prescribed quality standards and market demands the Indian Pharmaceutical Industry is under tremendous pressure to increase the extent and depth of implementation of Quality Assurance and Quality Management Systems (QMS), which require properly trained manpower.

During their experience in the execution of various consulting projects in pharmaceutical industry and in teaching the module on Quality Assurance and Quality Management Systems, the authors felt that there is a necessity to bring out a book with simple and lucid presentation of the basic concepts on QA and QMS.

The authors made a bold attempt in this book to present the basic concepts on various topics like QMS, GLP, GMP, Quality Audit, Statistical Quality Control and the analytical methods for QA. The elements, requirement and interpretation of ISO 9000 series of QMS are presented giving their origin and their precise role in management of quality of an international level of best practice.

The principles of GLP and GMP are discussed which are expected to guide the manufacturer and the regulator for maintaining high scientific and professional standards for ensuring only drugs of highest quality are produced and marketed. Further they also help the development of quality test data which forms the basis for the mutual acceptance of quality among countries and help to avoid the creation of technical barriers to trade and further help to improve the protection of human health and environment. Statistical Quality Control concept for improving the product quality are presented. These will greatly help for identification of factors responsible for decline in quality during initial stage of production and to take corrective measures and also helps in controlling the manufacture process more effectively. The various statistical tools used at both process control and product quality are discussed. The methods of analytical Quality Assurance presented in this book provide information and possible solutions of routine practice. Auditing is an important quality tool and is discussed with a basic framework of planning, conducting the audit, analysis of the results and reports and corrective actions. Each chapter is provided with a summary and typical questions which will be very useful in student's point of view.

This book is planned to cater to the needs of U.G/P.G students in pharmacy and Analytical chemistry and as a reference material for scientists and management personnel working in various pharmaceutical industries. For successful implementation of QA and QMS, the personnel need to have both technical and regulatory knowledge and should be able to apply in various situations with precise plans and actions following defined process and this book is aimed in presenting necessary guidelines in this direction.

In the appendix, the latest information on the International Standards of QMS, GLP and GMP are included for ready reference.

The authors thank Prof. K. Rajagopal, Vice Chancellor JNTU for writing foreword and Prof. C.K. Kokhate, Former Vice Chancellor Kakatiya University and Former President for Pharmacy Council of India for writing the Prologue. The authors also thank Prof. P. N Rao, Guest Faculty, JNT University for giving valuable suggestions and proof reading, Mr. P. V. Mukunda Rao, Mr. G. Sagareswar, Mr. Daniel and Mr. Vivek research students JNTU for their help in the preparation of the manuscript.

Authors

Y. Anjaneyulu

R. Marayya

Contents

Chapter 3
Good Laboratory Practice (GLP)

Chapter 4

Methods of Analytical Quality Assurance (AQA)

Chapter 5

Interpretation of Good Manufacturing Practice-Guide for Active Pharmaceutical Ingredients

Chapter 6

Statistical Quality Control

Chapter 7

Quality Audit

1

Introduction

1.0 Introduction

In today's context, "Quality" word is being used very frequently and in every situation. To an illiterate "Quality" means getting a real or maximum value to his money. To a civilian "Quality" means conforming to his requirements and serving the ultimate purpose.

'Thus, Quality is essential for survival and growth of any organization. Very oftenly, it signifies excellence of a product or service, which is measured upon the customer's actual experience with the product or service against his or her requirement. Quality is basically a customer's determination and hence, cannot be determined by producer or supplier'.

A quality management system organizes overall activities of the company in such a way that technical, administrative, and human factors affecting the quality of its products or services are under control. All such controls are oriented towards reduction, elimination and prevention of quality deficiencies.

The quality control systems consist of a defined set up and follow through operation to demonstrate assurance for Quality. The quality of design is the quality, which the manufacturer is intending to offer to the customer, and has the maximum influence on the quality of the product to be manufactured. Since design being the very first activity towards production it is essential that all inputs of design are accurately collected and reviewed at every stage inorder to make it a foolproof system.

The design and development of a process involves the translation of customer requirements in terms of product specification, material specification, process and service specification from which the various functions can perform these planned activities to produce the product of what the customer actually desires.

Inorder to get the desired quality, it is essential that all production operations, like process capability, production planning, material control, etc. are performed under controlled conditions and the Quality of the products is monitored by analysing the constituents by analytical Laboratories.

The ISO / IEC guide 25 has been adopted as a basis for establishing quality systems in analytical laboratories for recognizing their compliance through implementation of guidelines on general requirements for competent calibration and testing laboratory. The use of this guide will facilitate cooperation between laboratory and other bodies to assist in the exchange of information and experience and harmonization of standards and procedures. The guide also provides a mechanism for promoting confidence in calibration and testing laboratories, which demonstrate that they operate in accordance with the requirements for calibration and testing activities. Any new analytical procedure which required for validation before optimization of various individual steps verifying the entire fundamental analytical procedure for its performance in a given condition and its performance characteristics should be properly documented.

1.1 Quality Assurance and Quality Management in the Pharmaceutical Industry

Design, development and implementation of Quality assurance is the most vital function in the pharmaceutical industry. The skills necessary to optimally maintain such a vital function require additional technical capabilities and competence of the personnel who perform such a vital functional responsibilities. Hence, this function requires advanced training in several technical and scientific disciplines.

In Pharmaceutical industry, the Quality is a measure of a high degree of managerial, scientific and technical sophistication.

The control function (Quality control and Quality assurance) deals with acceptance and prevention activities. Quality assurance function deals with a system of management review of the performance and effectiveness of acceptance and prevention activities.

The Quality control and Quality assurance functions have been recognized as management tools and became a more formalized and systematized activity in the pharmaceutical industry. Today in the globalization scenario, due to global competition pressure, one need to be responsive to competitive requirements. As these requirements keep changing, inorder to meet customer's continuous changing requirements, supplier organization has to understand these requirements and must decide to change accordingly inorder to be in business. Inorder to meet such a challenge task and to improve business and establish growth in the business one has to understand and ensure that one really does what he claims to do, the first time and all the time. If we do what we really mean and faithfully try to serve, we do, not have to worry about anything else. The future has its own way of taking care of itself that is nothing but right system is built into the organization which will help to run the business profitably as the days proceed.

Total Quality philosophy has become an integral part of business management in different situations in the pharmaceutical industry. In the present context, " Quality" has become a buzz word and this word "Quality" is normally referred to "Conformance to specifications". This narrow definition of Quality, refers to inspection and servicing of products. This has been expanded to the service extended to customer to obtain customer satisfaction. The total Quality philosophy is a different way of managing business to gain maximum productivity, profitability and customer loyalty. This philosophy is extended to manage business in such a way that the customers are totally satisfied with the products and services as provided by the suppliers and finally this should be achieved at a low cost.

1.2 Quality Control

1.2.1 Quality Control in an Industry

The term "quality control" comprises of two words quality and control. Control is a universal regulatory process. In the industry, it takes the form of meeting standards. The process through which we establish and meet standards is called "control". This process has universal series of steps. Steps applied to problem of quality can be listed as follows :

- choosing the control subject, means what is to be regulated
- choosing an unit of measure
- setting a standard value, means of specifying quality characteristics
- providing a device which can measure the characteristics in terms of the unit of measure

- conducting actual measurements
- interpreting the difference between actual and standard
- taking decision and acting on the difference

When this universal regulatory process is applied to problems of product quality, it is called "quality control".

1.2.2 Quality Control in an Analytical Testing Laboratory

This refers to various operations that need to be undertaken in the laboratory to ensure that the data produced or generated will be of acceptable degree of accuracy and precision. The laboratory management must know the limits of accuracy of the data and hence, this should be the objective of Quality control. Inorder to achieve this objective, the Quality control function should take into consideration of various parameters like

- Trained manpower
- Use of appropriate laboratory standards
- Use of appropriate and calibrated instruments
- Laboratory data capture and details of data
- Safety in operations
- Laboratory analysis cost.

Unless, we consider these aspects scientifically, we cannot produce the product (Final Analytical report) with accuracy and low cost without which, Quality control function cannot be competitive. This aspect has not been taken very seriously in many Indian organisations.

1.3 Quality Assurance

Although Quality control function represents the core activity in Quality assurance programme, Quality assurance has a more major role to play than merely addressing technical aspects of Quality control. In the past, the words "Quality", "Quality control", and "Quality Assurance" have been used interchangeably without proper differentiation in the usage. The Japanese have taken triple concepts of Quality, reasonable price and mass production as business basics and succeeded in dominating the market in various fields of electronic, consumer goods, and automobiles. Further, Japanese have pioneered with the use of statistical principles necessary to control and assure quality in the manufacturing operations. We need to visualize analytical laboratory process also as a manufacturing process and assure that similar principles of Quality Control and assurance apply in the laboratory.

The series of testings performed to complete the analysis may be treated as a process and the resultant product is nothing but an analytical report. Fig. 1.1.

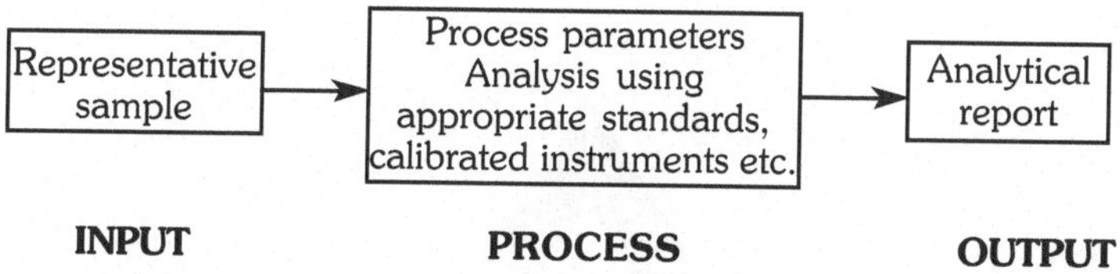

Figure 1.1 Analytical laboratory process for quality control.

The Quality refers to the accuracy of the output. For example in the laboratory, it refers to the analysis results, their accuracy and finally degree of management. Quality Assurance should design and develop a programme whereby Quality control laboratory can assure customers (Clients, customers, regulatory bodies etc.,) that the generated laboratory data is of proven quality.

Quality Assurance programme is a management tool and must assure the management that the activities are being performed as designed in all areas of operations within the organization. Inorder to achieve this goal effectively and efficiently, Quality Assurance team must commit to insist that every department to implement the following points :

- Selection of a concept of product or service to be responsive to the identified needs of the user.
- Different professionals in the field of quality have used different terms to designate the extent to which the intended features of the product respond to the actual market needs. Some of them are "Quality of concept", "Quality of project, Quality of design".
- Translation of selected concepts into a detailed set of specifications, when executed, will meet the needs of the user. The term "Quality of specifications" has been used to describe the extent to which the actual design specifications conform to the needs for fitness for use or for the grade.

The total progression of these activities is usually called the quality of design.

1.4 Triple Role Concept

Every unit of the organization-the entire company, each division, each department, each person-carries out process and produces a product. Such units may be called as Processor Team. Each processor team carries out three quality-related roles of (Fig. 1.2) the Customer, Processor and Supplier.

As a Customer, the processor team acquires various kinds of inputs from their suppliers, which are used in carrying out the process. The inputs may be in the form of materials, machineries, technology, methods, informations, services etc.

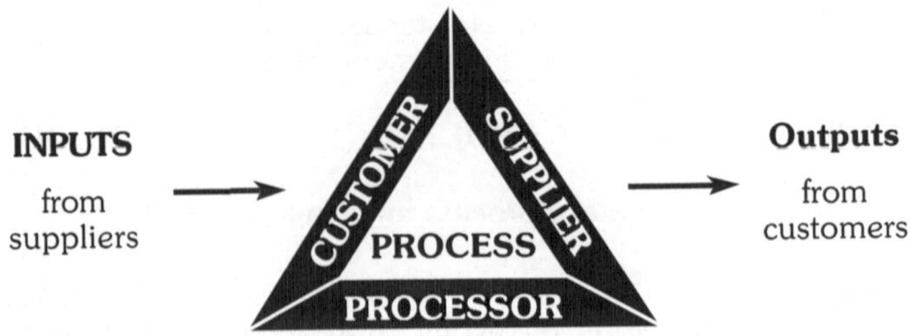

Figure 1.2 Triple role diagram.

1.5 Customer Requirement of Quality

Inorder to meet the customer requirements, every supplier has to understand the needs of customer, and every processor has to provide the required quality features in the product during its processing.

As a **Processor,** the processor team carries out various technological and managerial activities inorder to produce the product, which may be in the form of hardware, processed material, software or services.

As a **Supplier** the processor team supplies its products to its customers, who may be an internal customer or an external customer.

As shown in the following customer-supplier chain model (Fig. 1.3), each processor team is linked with its supplier and customer. Irrespective of whether the customer or supplier is an internal, belonging to own organization or an external one, the requirements must be met.

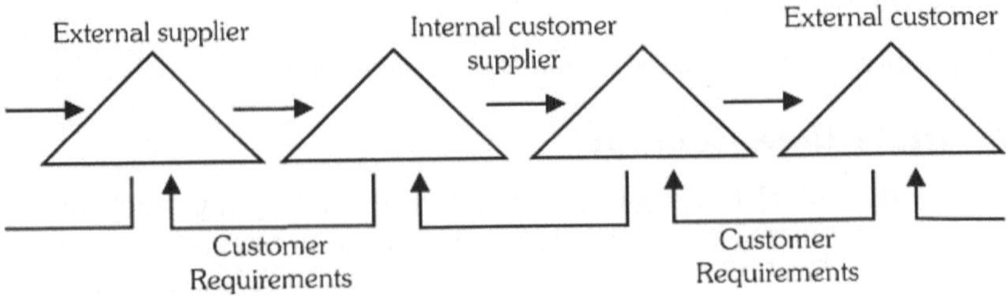

Figure 1.3 Customer-Supplier chain model.

Thus it is the responsibility of the supplier's management to provide adequate Quality Assurance to the customer. The quality assurance is "a planned and systematic activity operated by management to provide them with the confidence to meet the customer requirements". Thus implementation of ISO 9000 series of Quality Management system requirements assures your customers that you will provide acceptable and consistent Quality.

1.6 Quality Systems And Quality Management Systems

"Quality" is defined by customer needs and expectations, and it is also referred in several ways such as "fitness for use," "fitness for purpose", "customer satisfaction" or "conformance to requirements" etc., Though, these are only certain facets of quality, the complete explanation of quality leads to the definition of quality as "The totality of features and characteristics of product or service, that bear on it's ability, to satisfy stated or implied needs. In a simple and practical language we can say Quality as meeting the customer requirements".

1.6.1 Where from the 'Quality comes' ?

The quality comes from a process. A process is the transformation of a set of inputs, which can include actions, materials, methods and operations into desired outputs in the form of products, information, services or results are to be analyzed by examination of its inputs and outputs Fig. 1.4. This will determine the actions, which will be necessary to improve quality.

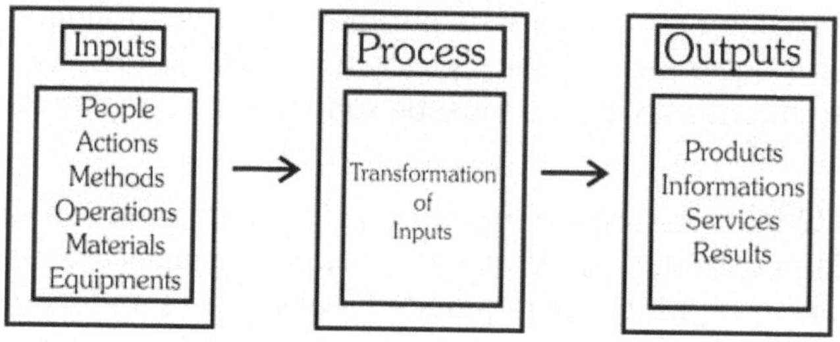

Figure 1.4 A process model.

The output of a process is transferred to somewhere or to someone- the customer. To produce an output, which meets the customer's requirements, it is essential to define, monitor and the control the inputs in the process and identify what constitutes fitness for use.

In a process function which influence the parameters responsible for fitness for use by the customer for any productive or activity depends on quality of design, quality of conformance, availability and field service as shown in Fig. 1.5.

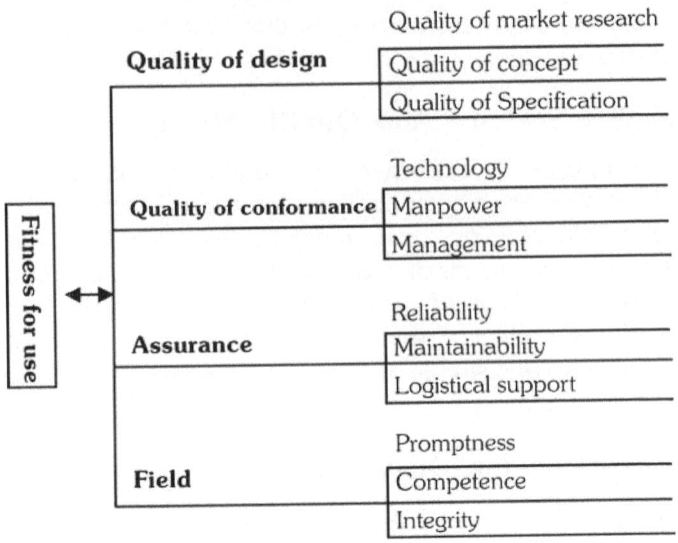

Figure 1.5 Fitness for use.

A difference in the quality of grade (which include level of fitness of the product for use and level of purchasing power of the customer) will determine the quality of design of the product.

The interrelation of the various parameters, which influence the level of fitness of the product for use, is shown in Fig.1.5. Procedures, record of the observations as required must be supervised during implementation phase.

A good Quality Assurance programme in an organization will not only have quality results but also prove that data is in place either to customer or regulatory authorities as required. Finally, this should be a positive assurance to management to achieve their goal in business and aim for business growth.

1.7 How to Achieve Quality?

Quality never happens by accident, it is always the result of an intelligent effort and therefore it has to be managed. Quality can be achieved through a quality management system, which must involve every one in the process throughout the organization.

A quality management system organizes overall activities of the company in such a way that the technical, administrative and human factors affecting the quality of its products or services are under control. All such controls are oriented towards the reduction, elimination and most importantly prevention of quality deficiencies.

The quality management system has to meet with the inter-related needs of the company as well as of the customer. The company's need is to attain and maintain desired quality at optimum cost by efficient utilization of it's technological, human and material resources. The customer will get confidence in the capability of company to deliver the desired quality product or service at competitive cost and maintain the same consistently.

The quality management system puts into practice the cost-effective concepts of getting it right first time, every time. The quality management starts with identification of customer needs and quality requirements and ends only when the product has been placed in the hands of customer who remains satisfied and ultimately should recommend to other customer.

The quality management system guides the co-ordinated actions of people, machines and information to achieve the quality objectives. ISO 9000 standards are intended to develop and establish a quality management system to accomplish the quality objectives of the company.

1.8 Quality Objectives

The concept of management of objectives is widely practised. Under this concept Manager participates in discussing objectives, and these become the basis for planning for results. These objectives are known as quality objectives. A well defined quality objective help managers thinking to stimulate action and permit comparison of performance against objectives. Objectives may be either for breakthrough or for control.

In small organizations, the chief executive by personal observation and by direct contact with the people can set quality objectives. In a large organization, this personal contact is no more feasible. There is no other alternative, except the leadership for setting quality objectives and the same is passed on to the departmental heads and thus, the quality objectives tend to be departmental rather than corporate. A large company can establish an interdepartmental mechanism to identify potential objectives, assess their economic and other effects and fix a priority in the programme of action.

The inputs, given below can help in identifying quality objectives:

- *Pareto analysis of repeated external alarm signals (e.g. complaints, returns etc.)
- Pareto analysis of repeated internal alarm signals (e.g. rejection, reprocessing etc.)
- Proposals from key persons in the organization i.e. managers, supervisors, professionals etc.
- Proposal from suggestion schemes.
- Data from field study of user's needs, costs;
- Comparison data on performance of the product versus competitor's product.
- Comments of key people outside organization i.e. customers, vendors, critics, press etc.
- Findings or comments of regulatory agency, independent laboratories or reformers.

A small note on Pareto principle will be helpful, Vilfredo Pareto an Italian economist had studied the distribution of wealth and had quantified the extent of inequality of this distribution. Although he had not generalized this concept of inequal distribution to other fields, but it was observed that the phenomenon of vital few and trivial many was universal. This phenomenon was later given the name of *Pareto Principle.

An objective is not likely to get priority unless it is quantified. Managers have multiple objectives for which they are accountable. Inview of this, advocate of specific objectives should get them quantified so that these get priority. Some typical statements of quantification are as follows : (Table 1.1)

Table 1.1 Quality objectives and qualified goals

Natural of objective	**Quantified goals**
Product improvement :	To make a tablet for with reduced disintegration time of less than one minute within three months
Training	To conduct GLP training for analysts within 30 days
Cost reduction	To reduce cost of packing material of product x by the first half of the financial year

1.9 Top Management Quality Approach

At the upper management level, quality objectives usually face competition from other objectives. Top management has strong bias with respect to three vital criteria.

- Top management prefers objectives for breakthrough over the objectives for control. The former has potential for long-range progress of the company while the latter is concerned with short term targets. Further, in the latter case, top management tries to delegate responsibility to lower level
- Top management exhibits a bias for projects of a business or management nature. Although technology is one of the means for meeting the business objectives, but not many top managers understand it prospectively.
- In the company, there are two common languages. At the bottom of the company that is below supervisors, foreman etc. the language is in terms of "things". Any one at this level talks, he talks about units of products, manhours or other materials or things.

For implementing the quality policy i.e. "Overall intentions and directions of an organization regarding quality as formally declared and authorized by the top management". The responsibility and commitment to quality should be reserved with the highest level of management. The top management may adopt various management techniques and styles to achieve quality objectives. The top management may consider the following actions.

1. Quality policy should be defined and declared.
2. Responsibility and authority of managers should be defined.
3. A quality system should be established.
4. Function of the quality system should be reviewed at regular intervals.
5. Representatives of the management should be appointed at appropriate levels
6. An internal verification system should be established.

1.10 Quality Policy

Every company has to formulate a quality policy on the following points : Which level of clientele constitutes the organizations market? This matter will have a bearing on the quality of design.

Has the organization to strive for quality leadership or competitiveness or just adequacy?

Has the organization been selling standard products or has it been selling a service in which the product is one of the ingredients of sale? This matter will have a bearing on conformance to specifications.

Has the organization to market its products on the basis of high reliability at higher initial price or lower reliability at lower initial price?

Whether the effort is to be made to optimize user's cost or manufacturer's cost?

Whether the abilities are to be quantified?

Whether the organization is to rely for its controls on systems or on people?

At which level quality planning is to be done?

Whether the supplier is to be put on the team?

Whether top management should participate in quality planning and assurance or these should be delegated to others?

When the organization grows to such an extent that it gets involved in multiple markets and products, no one set of quality policies can fit into its all activities, this problem can be solved by creating several levels of quality policy and one of the levels is corporate quality policy. A corporate quality policy consists of the following :

A statement of those policies which are company wide in nature and are binding on all company's units. The corporate quality policy usually states the following :

- the purpose of writing and publishing quality policies
- motherhood statement
- the minimal actions to be taken by the divisions of the company with respect to quality
- delegation of authority to divisions to establish subsidiary quality policies appropriate to their requirements
- if required, quality policies for functional organization units or for programmed activities

While deciding and writing policy, following points may be considered :

- the policy should be relevant to the organization, its products and people;
- the objectives should be ambitious but achievable
- the policy should be practical in approach and realistic
- the policy should be written in easy and understandable language

In the process of formulating policies, the key managers should participate. However, they may not do detailed staff work. One way of doing this is to assign to a specialist the job of obtaining from these key managers the following :

- their nominations as to what should be the subject matter of quality policies
- their judgment as to the direction of company towards these subjects

Through this method, it is possible to find out consensus among these key managers on the identified subjects. A draft can be prepared based on the consensus which can be further discussed for finalizing the policies.

The top managers are responsible for product fitness for use and they are accountable to the directors, owners, regulators, public etc. These top managers can and often do delegate responsibility to subordinate managers for carrying out the activities that make up the quality function but they cannot delegate the accountability.

Until 1960s, examples of written quality policy were rare. Thereafter the number is increasing and the increase is likely to continue. While the written quality policy is mainly for internal use but broader publications may be necessary in view of the growing competition. Advantages of written policy are :

- it makes those concerned with it to think in depth as it can be written only after giving a thought
- written policy can be communicated in an authoritative manner
- it provides a basis for management by agreed policies rather than by crisis or opportunity
- audit of adherence to the policy can be done.

Before the policy is published, there should be a firm determination to adhere to it. If there is any doubt in adherence to it, it should not be published. Because in the long run, both insiders and outsiders draw their conclusions about the policy from the deeds of the company. If people see innovative products one after the other from a company, they conclude that the company has policy of design leadership. If a company attends to quality complaints promptly, the observer will conclude that company has policy of ethical dealing on quality. If the deeds of the company are in line with the policy, the written policy gains credibility. If written policy says something and deeds demonstrate something else, not only written policy of the company loses its credibility but other promises made by the company are looked at suspiciously.

1.11 What is ISO 9000?

The ISO 9000 is a series of five individual but inter-related standards on Quality Management & Quality Assurance Systems, which can be adopted by all types of organizations producing and supplying all kinds of goods, services or software. These standards are generic, not specific to any particular product, and can be used by manufacturing and service industries alike.

These standards were developed with the goal of effectively documenting the quality system elements to be implemented inorder to maintain an efficient quality system in an organization. The ISO 9000 standards do not themselves specify the technology to be used for implementing the quality system elements.

Implementation of ISO 9000 quality system guides in building quality into the product or services by prevention of quality deficiencies and imparts consistence quality.

The quality system applies to and interacts with all activities related to quality of a product or service. It can be explained through quality loop (Fig. 1.6.).

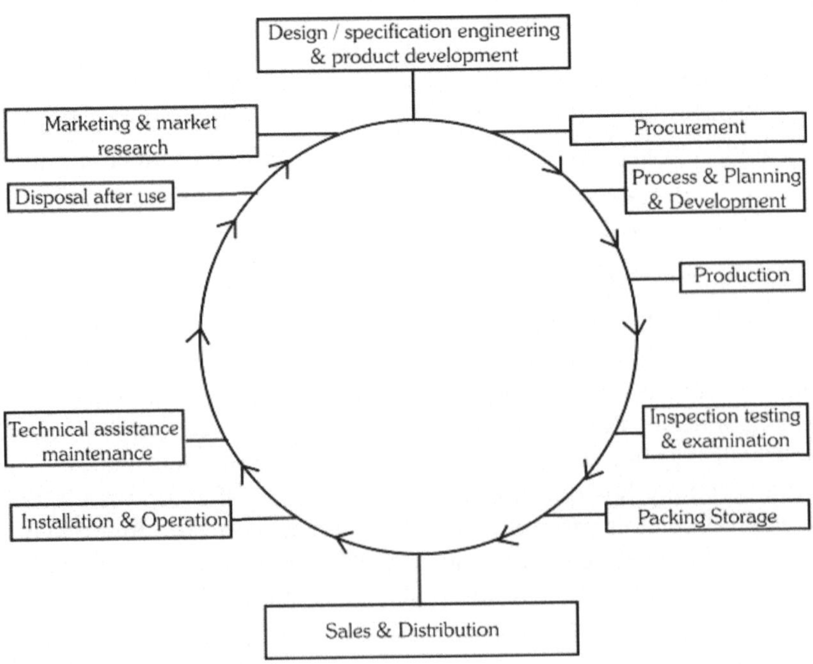

Figure 1.6 Quality loop.

The quality system involves all phases from initial identification to final satisfaction of requirements and expectations of customer.

Relationships of various activities can also be explained through the spiral of progress in quality. Achievements of fitness for use involve a number of separate deeds and activities in a logical progression. The main activities in the progression have been shown in the spiral of progress. A turn of the spiral of progress commences with product research and development to create an improvement in fitness for use, the object. At the end of that turn, the experience of user may create a new idea, which will start a new turn of the spiral for improvement. (Fig.1.7.).

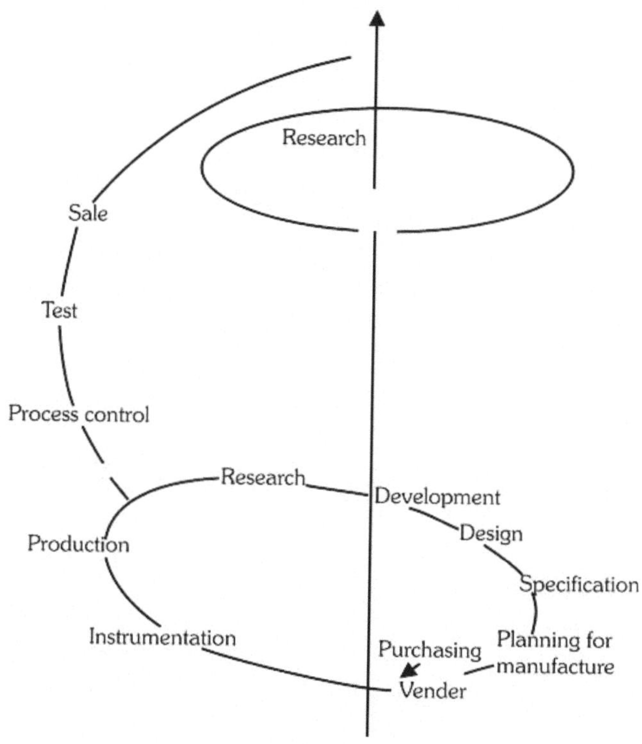

ISO 9001 : 2000 QMS Spiral to be incorporated

Figure 1.7 The spiral of progress in quality.

It may be seen from the spiral of progress in quality that activities needed to achieve the object, fitness for use, are scattered among several persons in several specialized departments.

It may also be seen that some departments are in- house and some are not. The outside persons are a part of supplies companies, merchant companies, user companies and consumer families. In certain companies, the specialized departments are also concerned with certain other functions, for example, cost, delivery, personnel, and technology. From this it can be very well made out that these departments have multiple goals as well. Today this is a major problem how to make them conducive to each other or to orchestrate them. These widely scattered activities constitute quality function. Thus quality function can be defined as the entire collection of activities through which we achieve fitness for use, no matter where these activities are performed.

Summary

Quality : Quality signifies excellence of a product or service, which is measured, based on customer's experience with the product or service against his or her requirements.

Quality control : Quality control deals with a system which accepts or rejects any activities which effect the Quality and prevents Quality deficiency and imparts consistency in the quality of the product or service.

Quality assurance : It is quality management (tool) system which organizes overall activities of the company or industry or organization in such a way that technical, administrative and human factors and assures the management that all the activities are being performed as designed in the organization.

Quality assurance in pharmaceutical industry : It is a measure of high degree of managerial, scientific, technical functions by sophisticated design and development. Implementation of quality assurance is the most vital function of total quality management in pharmaceutical industry and is considered as an internal part of business and market.

Triple role concept of quality management : It deals with the process or team which demands Quality related role from customers process or and supplier.

Customer-Suppler chain model : Each processor intern is linked with supplier-customer irrespective of whether this belongs to internal or external. The management has to ensure Quality assurance to the customer by implementing various Quality Management systems.

Process model for quality control : Determines the actions to be taken to improve the Quality, based on the implementation of a process which involves transformation of actions (which include actions, materials methods and operations) into a desired output.

Fitness for use of product quality : Depends on Quality of design, quality of conformance of product and/or service.

Quality objectives : For any industry or organization functional objectives should be well defined and quantified. It helps management to stimulate action and allow companies to perform against defined objectives. A large company has to establish an interdepartmental mechanism to identify important objectves of the company/ organization which need to work, assess their economic and other efforts and fix priorities of actions.

Quality polices and approach of top management : Every company has to formulate a well defined Quality polices and committment of top management. The responsibility of implementation of quality policy of the organization should be with the highest level of management.

ISO 9000 : is a series of five individual but interrelated Quality Management and Quality Assurance systems that can be adopted by all types of organizations.

Quality loop : It is a tool to understand the interactions of all activities in a Process which relate to Quality.

Spiral process in quality : It is a method to various depict validation of the independent activities in a particular process which are to be carried in a logical precision and quality product to meet standards of fitness for use by the customer.

This will help in better understanding between interrelated activities which effect the quality of the product and creation of new industries to better the quality of the product.

Questions

1. Explain the terms Quality, Quality control, Quality assurance with reference to total quality management in an industry?
2. What is Triple role concept and customer–supplier model in Quality Management?
3. Explain how the process Model for Quality control helps in describing the action to be taken to improve the Quality of a Product?
4. Discuss various factors, which effect fitness for use of the product Quality?
5. What is the importance of framing the quality policy and Quality objectives for any industry or organization?
6. Discuss the role of Quality policy and Management approach in Total Quality Management?
7. Discuss in brief about ISO 9000 series of Quality Management and Quality assurance standards?
8. Explain the use of Quality Loop and Spiral loop of process model in Quality assessment system?

2

Elements, Requirements and Interpretation of ISO 9001 : 2000 Quality Management System

2.1 Introduction and Historical Perspectives

The ISO 9000 Quality system is a series of international standards on quality management and quality assurance system, which can be adopted by all types of organizations producing and supplying all kinds of goods, services, software etc.,

ISO 9000 series constitute ISO 9000, 9001,9002,9003 and 9004.

ISO 9001, 9002, 9003, are three quality system models for external quality assurance. ISO 9001 is the most comprehensive-standard covering the design, manufacturing, installation and servicing systems, ISO 9002 covers manufacturing and installation and ISO 9003 covers only final product inspection and test. These three models were developed for use in contractual situations such as those between a customer and a supplier.

ISO 9004 provides guidelines for internal use by a manufacturer developing its own quality system to meet the business needs.

To attain ISO 9000 registration, a manufacturer must provide objective evidence that its management is actively involved in its quality process, that its participation with suppliers and customer is designed to ensure that all mutually determined requirements are understood and consistently met and that the text of the company's internal procedures ensures that serious attention is given to customer service and product quality.

The ISO 9000 standards also require that a company maintain control of its documented procedures that describe its methods for design, production, inspection, handling, storage and delivery of all materials and products as well as defining the system, that assures continuous employee training and development.

ISO 9000 standards are practical standards for quality management systems that can be applied by all types of business. They have found wide application as a basis for agreement between buyers and suppliers. The standards are based on two main foundations.

Management responsibility and commitment to quality, which should be expressed in formal policy statement and implemented through, appropriate measures.

A set of requirements that deal with each aspect of the company activity and organisation that affects quality.

An important condition for conformance to the standards is appropriate documentation of the quality policy and procedures, which put together form the quality Manual of the company. The evaluation of ISO 9000 series are schematically represented in Fig. 2.1 (a) while the overview of ISO 9000 series of standards are presented schematically in Fig. 2.1 (b).

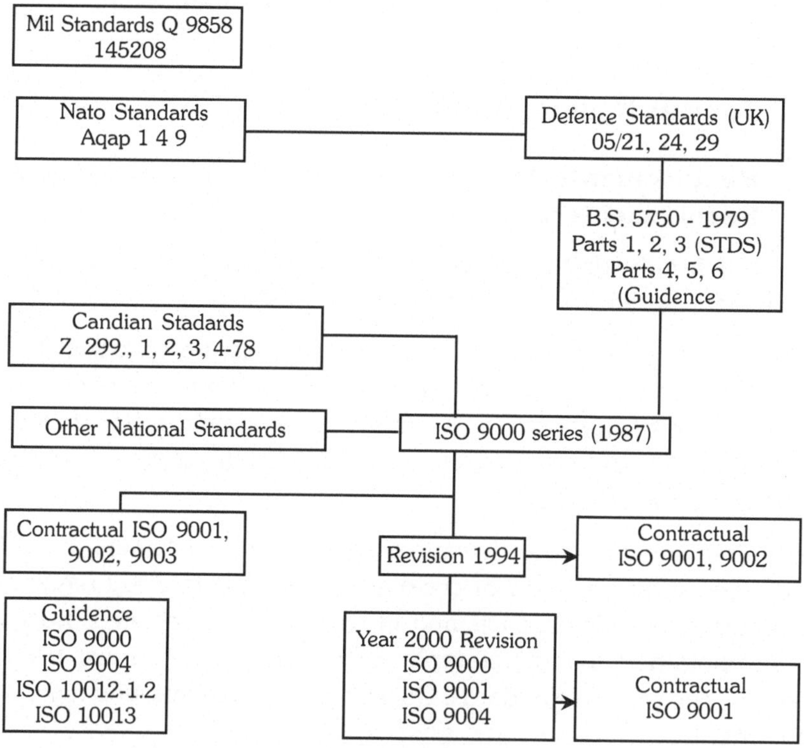

Figure 2.1 (a) Evolution of ISO 9000 series.

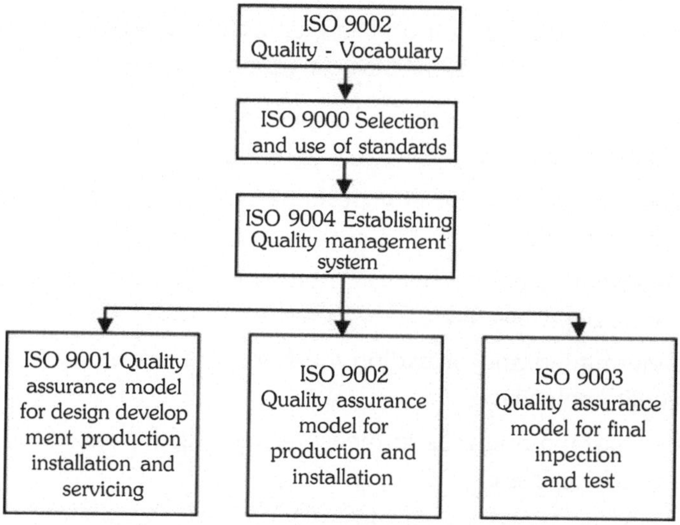

Figure 2.1 (b) Overview of ISO 9000 series of standards.

The elements of ISO 9001: 2000 quality assurance are given in appendix 1.

2.2 General Requirements

2.2.1 Requirements for Quality Management System and Requirements for Products

ISO 9000 family distinguishes between requirements for quality management systems and requirements for products.

Requirements for quality management systems are specified in ISO 9001. Requirements for quality management systems are generic and applicable to organization in any industry or economic sector regardless of the offered product category. ISO 9001 itself does not establish requirements for products.

Requirements for products can be specified by customers or by the organization in anticipation of customer requirements or by regulation. The requirements for products and in some cases associated processes can be contained in, for example, technical specifications, product standards, and process standards. Contractual agreements, and regulatory requirements.

2.2.2 Quality Management Systems (QMS) Approach

An approach for developing and implementing a quality management system consists of several steps including the following :

(a) Determining the needs and expectations of customers and other interested parties;

(b) Establishing the quality policy and quality objectives of the organization,

(c) Determining the processes and responsibilities necessary to attain the quality objectives;

(d) Determining and providing the resources necessary to attain the quality objectives;

(e) Establishing methods to measure the effectiveness and efficiency of each process;

(f) Applying these measures to determine the effectiveness and efficiency of each process;

(g) Determining means of preventing nonconformities and eliminating their causes :

(h) Establishing and applying a process for continually improving the existing management practices.

The following are general requirements for ISO 9000 both by QMS approach and Process approach

An organization that adopts the QMS or process approach creates confidence in the capability of its processes and the quality of its products, and provides a basis for continual improvement. This can lead to increased satisfaction of customers than other interested parties and to the success of the organization.

The following are general requirements for ISO 9000 either by process approach or QMS approach.

2.2.3 The Process Approach

Any activity, with a set of activities that uses resources to transform inputs to outputs can be considered as a process.

For organisations to function effectively, they have to identify and manage numerous interrelated and interacting processes. Often, the output from one process will directly form the input into the next process. The systematic identification and management of the processes employed within an organization and particularly the interactions between such processes are referred to as the "Process approach".

The intent of this international standard is to encourage the adoption of the process approach to manage an organization.

Fig. 2.2 illustrates the process based quality management systems as described in the ISO 9000 family of standards. The illustration shows that interested parties play a significant role in providing inputs to the organization. Monitoring the satisfaction of interested parties requires the evaluation of information relating to the perception of interested parties to the extent to which their needs and expectations have been met. The model shown in Figure 2.2 does not show processes at a detailed level but at a basic level.

In order to obtain registration, a company's quality system has to be continually assessed by an accredited third party / assessment agency.

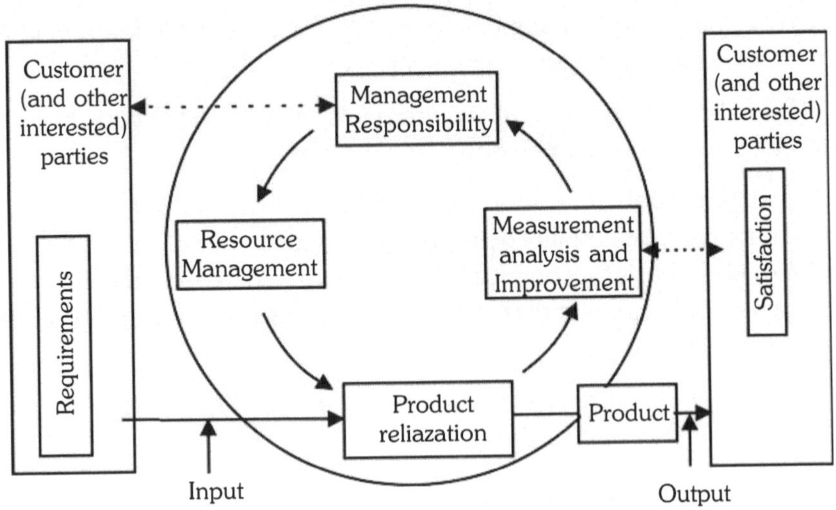

Figure 2.2 Continual improvement of the quality management system - process based.

2.2.4 QMS Approach Requirements

1. The supplier organization should establish, document, implement, monitor and continuously improve the effectiveness of the quality management system, (QMS) that should fulfill the requirements of the international QMS as per ISO 9001: 2000.
2. The organization should adopt a process approach in all areas of activities throughout the organization.
3. The responsible personnel of all departments should identify the processes in each department and establish the interactions with support functions within the identified process.
4. The key personnel should mobilise and ensure the availability of resources and information flow required to operate and monitor the progress within the process.
5. Identify the process parameters and justify the acceptance criteria.

6. Establish the methods of monitoring during operation and implementation of the process.
7. Regularly monitor and measure the processes, analyse these processes periodically inorder to establish that the identified processes are effective.
8. Organization should demonstrate that the identified processes are effective in yielding the desired results to achieve Organisation goals and to ensure continual improvement.

2.3 Documentation Requirements

2.3.1 General Requirements

The supplier Organisation should develop Quality Management System documentation based on the process approach concept and should be sound like a pyramid (Fig. 2.3). At the same time, the Organisation should develop documentation on need based approach and should ensure that every process shall be carefully planned, effective in operation and under control.

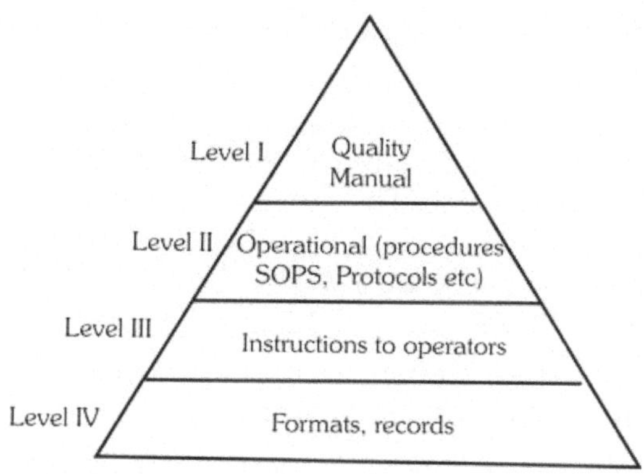

Figure 2.3 Documentation pyramid.

Thus, the Organisation structure can be suitably designed in four levels as shown above based on the Organisation size and its activities. Occasionally, smaller Organisation can combine level-II and level-III activities.

The key documentation should include :

(a) Quality policy statement and quality objectives, which are a means to achieve the quality policy.
(b) Quality manual.

(c) Operational procedures and instructions for each line of activity identified by the Organisation.

(d) The formats, which are a means to record the data.

(e) The records (quality), which are the tools to demonstrate the implementation status of organisation activities.

(f) The documentation can be either a manuscript or an electronic type.

2.3.2 Quality Manual

The Quality manual, which is a level-I document of the Organisation to include policy statements and should address all the elements / requirements specified in ISO-9001: 2000 guidance document.

A typical Quality Manual should be 25 to 30 A_4 size papers excluding the support data annexures where applicable.

The key requirement /principle underlying the development of Quality Manual should be

(a) It should address all the clauses of ISO-9001: 2000 QMS requirements. Where applicable, Organisation can claim exclusions of any clause with proper justification.

(b) The Organisation should define and document every applicable activity of each department, as a process and process map need to be described indicating possible interaction with support functions as applicable. The process flow map should be a guiding tool to achieve the objective of the defined process and further this should include the responsibilities and accountability of the personnel involved.

(c) The Organisation should establish and refer all the applicable procedures in the Quality Manual.

(d) The list of applicable records should be included.

2.3.3 Control of Documents

The Organisation should establish a single documented procedure to detail the structure of a procedure and/or work instruction.

The documented procedure should be a key document of the Organisation on which the entire documentation structure is based.

This key document should address the following but not limited to :

(a) The purpose or objective

(b) The scope

(c) The responsibility for preparation, review and approval. Additionally, the responsibility and accountability of personnel to implement the same.

(d) The activity description.

(e) The definitions of new terms and reference documents as applicable.

(f) The unique identification number, current revision status and review status.

(g) The list of formats for recording the status of activity.

(h) The review history and change history.

(i) The identification of the document status.

(j) The distribution list for the documents.

(k) The document should be legible, identifiable and ensure that the current document is at the point of use.

(l) The mechanism through which the obsolete documents are removed from the place of use as applicable and ensure that the recent version will be available at the point of use.

(m) The mechanism of destroying the obsolete documents and

(n) The list of external documents as applicable should be available and should include the mechanism through which such documents are controlled.

2.3.4 Control of Records

Primarily, a document can form a record when filled with the data. Record is an evidence of implementation or conformity to the requirements specified in the process. Thus, a record is the proof of implementation status and hence, should not be tampered.

(a) Records should be legible

(b) Bear unique identification

(c) Storage location and protection

(d) Storage period

(e) Accessibility status

(f) Disposal mechanism

(g) Easy retrieval as and when required

2.4 Management Responsibility

2.4.1 Role of Top Management Within the Quality Management System

Through leadership and actions, top management can create an environment where people are fully involved and in which a quality management system can operate effectively. The quality management principles can be used by top management as the basis of its role, which is as follows :

(a) To establish and maintain the quality policy and quality objectives of the organization;

(b) To promote the quality policy and quality objectives throughout the organization to increase awareness, motivation and involvement;

(c) To ensure focus on customer requirements throughout the organization;

(d) To ensure that appropriate processes are implemented to enable requirements of customers and other interested parties to be fulfilled and quality objectives to be achieved;

(e) To ensure that an effective land efficient quality management system is established, implemented and maintained.

(f) To achieve the quality objectives;

(g) To ensure the availability of necessary resources;

(h) To decide on actions regarding the quality policy land quality objectives.

(i) To decide on actions for improvement of the quality management system.

2.4.2 Management Commitment

Top management, which includes proprietor, owner and / or person responsible for business growth, should provide commitment with conviction to develop QMS system and implement and continually improve the effectiveness of implementation through an effective internal audit system.

Top Management should involve in the following activities but not limited to, :

(a) Identification of customers and business partners (suppliers)

(b) To release Quality policy and objectives document

(c) To draw road map to achieve the Quality objectives through effective management reviews.

(d) To provide the resources (technological, infrastructure, personnel, facilities and financial).

(e) To identify and document statutory and regulatory requirements.

2.5 Customer Focus

(a) To bring awareness in the Organisation with regard to the importance of customer and their requirements.

(b) To design an action plan to develop customers and achieve customer satisfaction.

(c) To facilitate promoting the concept of developing an internal customer relationship within the Organisation.

(d) To emphasize that every employee of the Organisation must develop and maintain customers within their own field of activity and finally to achieve 'customer delight'.

2.6 Quality Policy Document

Quality Policy and Quality Objectives :

Quality policy and quality objectives are established to provide a focus to direct the organization. Both determine the desired results and assist the organization to apply its resources to achieve these results. The quality policy provides a framework for establishing and reviewing quality objectives. The quality objectives need to be consistent with the quality policy and the commitment to continual improvement, and their achievement needs to be measurable. The achievement of quality objectives can have a positive impact on product quality, operational effectiveness and financial performance and thus on the satisfaction and confidence of interested parties.

Top Management person should release the Quality policy and objectives document.

The Quality policy document should be framed keeping inview of organization's.

(a) Vision, Mission and policy matters to sustain and develop business.

(b) Commitment to comply with statutory and regulatory requirements as well as customer's requirements.

(c) Commitment to develop and implement QMS to achieve business objectives.

(d) Commitment to continually improve upon QMS implementation to achieve customer delight and business prosperity.

(e) Facilitate the employees to build and adopt "Quality work culture" as a walk of life.

2.7 Planning

2.7.1 Quality Objectives

The Top Management team should frame the quality objectives, which are a means to achieve the Quality Policy. These Quality objectives should be appropriate for organisation's overall performance.

The key points to be considered while framing the Quality objectives are :

(a) To develop Quality Human resource.
(b) To understand current and future market demands/ requirements.
(c) To understand the product requirements of customers.
(d) To achieve satisfaction of customers through quality supplies.
(e) To continually improve upon the performance of the processes.
(f) To provide necessary and appropriate resources to facilitate Quality supplies and win-over customer.
(g) To identify and achieve opportunities for improvement.
(h) Periodical assessment of organisation results.
(i) Periodical reviews to understand the current status and improve upon the practices continually.

2.8 Responsibility, Authority and Communication

2.8.1 Responsibility

Top management should frame and release a document titles "Organisation Chart" which should include the reporting hierarchy in the Organisation. The responsibilities and authorities of personnel should be documented. The responsibilities of personnel need to be defined explicitly and should be communicated to all personnel within the Organisation.

2.8.2 Management Representative (MR)

Top management should identity a key person within the Organisation to act as a representative to monitor the implementation of QMS on continual basis. This representative will be normally represented by the term "Management Representative" (MR).

The Management Representative should be a senior position in the Organisation, knowledgeable, communicative, and should be capable of leading the team for achieving business results.

Generally, the Management Representative should have the following additional responsibilities.

(a) To ensure establishment of QMS requirements, to facilitate implementation and maintain continually.

(b) To ensure propagation of customer's requirements among all employees.

(c) To ensure effective implementation of QMS through effective internal audit system.

(d) To report the overall status of performance of QMS to Top Management periodically.

(e) To identify the areas for improvement.

(f) To liaison with external parties as and when required.

2.8.3 Internal Communication

The internal communication requirement is essential and necessary in any Organisation. This area is by and large has not been taken in spirit. This should include the mechanism through which the company's Policies, procedures, customer's requirements, customers remarks etc are made known to relevant personnel within the Organisation.

2.9 Management Review

"Management Review" as this term sounds should include the review of activities within the Organisation by the Management at defined intervals inorder to understand the current status and assess opportunities to achieve business goals. This is defined as a "process".

2.9.1 Review INPUT

The input items for Management Review should include but not limited to :

(a) Quality policy and objectives status

(b) Customers requirements and feedback.

(c) Internal audit results

(d) Status of effectiveness of corrective actions and preventive actions taken

(e) Product and process requirements

(f) Resources requirements

(g) Changes that affect QMS

(h) Scope and recommendations for improvement
(i) Follow-up actions of previous management review.

2.9.2 Review Output

Should include Management's decision based on review

(a) QMS Improvement requirements
(b) Customers requirements
(c) Resource requirements
(d) Product/Process requirements

2.9.3 Process

(a) Conducting management review to discuss input items
(b) Should include all departmental Heads as members of the group.
(c) Management review report preparation and submission to Top Management by MR.

2.10 Resource Management

2.10.1 Provision of Resources

The Organisation should establish a procedure to define the methodology to provide the necessary resources, which include

- Technological Resource
- Facility Resource
- Infrastructure resource
- Human Resource
- Business development resource

The required resources need to be identified through Management review process.

The Top management should ensure its commitment to continually improve upon the effectiveness of QMS.

2.10.2 Human Resources

2.10.2.1 General Requirement

In general and by and large in batch processing operation industry, and in semi-automatic industry, the human resource play a key and vital role in producing consistent Quality of product and/ or service.

Hence, for this reason, the personnel involved in the manufacturing industry should be competent, based on education, training, skills and experience.

2.10.2.2 Competence, Awareness and Training

The Organisation should ensure that

(a) The personnel involved in the operation are aware of their role and importance in producing consistent Quality Product.

(b) The personnel are responsible to contribute their mite in achieving the Quality objectives.

(c) The personnel are competent in their activity. Competency can be defined as application of knowledge and skills to the extent required.

Knowledge : Through appropriate education and Qualification.

Skills : Through appropriate training

Competence : Application of Knowledge and Skills

Hence, training of personnel is a must to upgrade their skills and competency levels.

(d) The personnel are evaluated periodically for their knowledge, skills and attitude towards work.

(e) The evaluation of personnel are carried out for the effectiveness of training programmes provided through examination, group discussion, performance improvement in their activity after training etc.,

(f) To maintain employees records which include details of education, experience, training, competency levels, and evaluation status on continuous basis. Generally, these training records are permanent till the employees serve in the industry.

2.10.3 Infrastructure Resource

The organisations management should provide adequate infrastructure resource required to achieve product specific requirements and customer's additional requirements.

The infrastructure resource include the following.

- Building facility with appropriate design meeting the standards.

- Equipment and utilities
- Adequate green belt to maintain the environments
- Conduce work environment in the facility

2.11 Product Realisation

2.11.1 Planning of Product Realisation

The Organisation should plan and develop the process for product realisation. The Organisation should develop a document, usually referred to as "Quality plan" that should be applied either product based or project based.

Facility	:	Verification and validation report
Equipment	:	Inspection, qualification and testing record
Process document	:	Product acceptance record
		Customer satisfaction record

2.11.2 Customer Related Processes

2.11.2.1 Determination of requirements related to the product

The Organisation should document a procedure to develop and maintain customers base who are the purpose of the business. The purpose of the business includes maintaining the current customers and develops the new customers to sustain in business and to promote growth in the Organisation. This phase basically speaks of the marketing and sales department functionality. The Organisation should develop a procedure, which should capture the following requirements about the product.

(a) Receipt of customers requirements with regard to product Quality specifications and commercial terms specifications.

(b) The terms pertaining to delivery, post delivery activities

(c) The provision to discuss with the customers with regard to the intended use of the product

(d) The statutory and regulatory requirements.

(e) Any additional requirements that will be determined by the Organisation to improve upon the use of the product.

(f) The receipt of requirements can be verbal, hard copy, or electronic form.

2.11.2.2 Review of requirements related to the product

The Organisation should review the requirements before the Organisation offers commitment to the customer. This review should ensure the review of functional characteristics of the product by Quality department and commercial.

(a) Product specifications receipt and review by quality department.

(b) To decide the organization's ability to meet with the requirements.

(c) Communication to management with the regard to the ability of the Organisation to meet with the customer's requirements.

(d) If any issue is to be resolved, the Organisation should communicate to the customer and the issues should be resolved prior to acceptance of the order.

(e) The customer specified requirements should be treated as final.

2.11.2.3 Customer communication

(a) This phase refers to the communication part of the process with the customer.

(b) Before communication with the customer the organization should ensure the documents, pertaining to the receipt, review and amendment where necessary of the customer product / supply requirements.

(c) Any additional commercial terms as applicable.

(d) Convert the enquiry into formal order.

(e) Acceptance of the order by the organization.

(f) Supply the product as per the agreed terms and conditions.

(g) Monitor the supply position and communicate to the customer any delay as and when applicable.

(h) Permanent records should be maintained by the organization.

2.12 Designs and Development

This phase of study refers to Research and Development function in the organization. This activity is applicable to new product and/or process discovery and/or existing product process modifications or changes as applicable. Hence this process detail of the total development activity phase, which can be divided into sub activates in the product cycle.

2.12.1 Design and Development Planning

The organization should ensure the following :

(a) The top management should identify the areas /product to be considered for development.

(b) Internal communication with the R&D function.

(c) The organization should ensure to develop a procedure, which should chronologically capture the details and methodology, such as identification of product, literature search, product feasibility study, development phase. Identification of materials, their characteristics at different phases of study during optimization of process, validation of process, stability and safety studies of the product, scale up studies plan and preparation of a formal development report.

(d) The procedure should capture the responsibilities and authorities of personnel at each stage of design and development.

(e) The interface communication scheme with different functions / groups and their responsibilities need to be clearly defined and documented.

(f) The organization should ensure to establish a document, which deals with all the activities of validations "Master Validations Plan".

2.12.2 Design and Development Input

The R & D development should define and ensure the following :

(a) Product characteristics.

(b) Safety, statutory and regulatory requirements.

(c) Information on experimental design.

(d) Materials and facilities which include testing.

(e) Trained manpower.

(f) Laboratory notebooks to capture the online information.

2.12.3 Design Development Outputs

The design and development review out put documents should consider the following :

(a) The testing results of the product.

(b) The yield / out put quantity of the product.

(c) The inference /conclusions for each experiment out put review.

2.12.4 Design and Development Review

This phase of study should consider the following :

(a) Evaluation of the test result and product quality against the documented specifications.

(b) Identification of problems encountered.

(c) Proposal for future experiments and define the scope.

(d) Conclusions to be drawn based on the review.

2.12.5 Design and Development Verification

This phase of study should include the following :

(a) Optimization of process characteristics preferably through statistical experimental design patterns.

(b) Identification of critical process parameters and fixing the tolerance criteria.

(c) Justification of tolerance criteria based on experimental data.

(d) Identification and justification of in-process quality checks and their tolerance limits.

(e) Justification of out put yield range values.

(f) Identification of measuring instruments review for calibration.

(g) Thorough review of out put product against the specified input requirements.

(h) Document the details of investigations and prepare a final report.

2.12.6 Design and Development Validation

Validation : This is a process through which one need to establish documented evidence that a product /process will consistently produce quality product which ensures meeting with the pre defined acceptance criteria. During this phase of validation study, the following activities need to be planned and carried out.

(a) The master validation plan document

(b) Facilities validation

(c) Qualification of equipments

(d) Calibration of measuring instruments

(e) Qualification of input materials

(f) Product quality specification and test methods

(g) Method validation

(h) Process validation

(i) Equipment cleaning method validation
(j) Trained man power and competency of personnel
(k) Stability studies data evaluation
(l) Validation report at each phase of validation study.

2.12.7 Control of Design and Development Changes

In any process, deviations are inevitable when a deviation is encountered, the deviation need to be investigated and documented. During the process of investigation, certain changes are required to be incorporated to salvage the product or modification of the process. Hence, as deviation is inevitable so is the change too.

When changes are to be made, these changes are to be verified and to be ratified.

In this phase of study, the organization should ensure the following :

(a) Document the deviations
(b) Failure investigation process
(c) Handling of non –conformity product
(d) Handling of change controls
(e) Handling of Customer complaints
(f) Handling of product recall
(g) Handling of returned product

2.13 Purchasing

2.13.1 Purchasing Process

The organization should ensure the conformity of the materials with the established specifications. The organization should evaluate the implication of these purchased materials on the finished product manufactured by the organization. The quality of the finished product hence depends upon the quality of the input materials supplied either through manufacturers or suppliers. Hence, the need indirectly is on the quality of the suppliers and/or original manufacturers.

In order to control the quality of input materials, which is an essential requirement should, consider the following phases.

(a) The selection of suppliers for input materials.
(b) The supply of documented specifications to the suppliers.
(c) The acceptance from the suppliers to meet the requirements.

(d) The commercial aspects such as cost, delivery schedules, transportation, and post delivery aspects are part of the requirements and need to be addressed and sorted out between suppliers and organization prior to start of supplies.

(e) The technical evaluation of materials by the organization for compliance of input materials specifications.

(f) The organization should evolve a policy for evaluation of suppliers based on quality characteristics and other commercial terms (hidden requirements).

(g) The organization should develop a procedure, which should address selection, evaluation, continuous monitoring, periodical reevaluation and deleting of non-quality suppliers.

(h) The records should be maintained for all these activities to demonstrate its effective implementation.

Hence, in today's business scenario, suppliers hold the real key/success of an organizations business and hence they are to be treated as business partners.

2.13.2 Purchasing Information

In order to control the quality of input materials and their suppliers, the organization should provide the following required information to the suppliers prior to procurement.

(a) Requirements for product quality (Grade, type, class etc.,)

(b) Documented specifications / drawing as applicable.

(c) Quality specifications and price.

(d) Type of packing and delivery schedules.

(e) Inspection details as applicable.

(f) Other relevant commercial terms.

(g) Statutory requirements.

Hence, to provide these information to the suppliers prior to release of purchase Order is an essential requirement and such responsibility lies on the part of the organization.

2.13.3 Verification of Purchased Product

The organization should evolve a policy document for verification/ inspection process of the purchased product. This inspection process include:

(a) Inspection of input materials by the organization in their premises.

(b) Inspection of input materials by the organization at the supplier's location prior to release of materials where applicable.

(c) Inspection of input materials at the supplier's place prior to release by the organization's representative.

(d) Receipt of supplies COA along with the consignment and verification of these results by the organization's COA (certificate of analysis).

(e) This inspection process is applicable to contact manufacture operations also.

2.14 Production and Service Operations

This requirement/process deals with the various activities that are needed to be performed in the manufacturing which cover the following :

(a) Production process and service operations

(b) Validation of applicable processes

(c) Materials identification, storage and traceability

(d) Customers property/material

(e) Packaging and delivery of the product

(f) Monitoring and measuring devices control and calibration.

2.14.1 Control of Production and Service Operations

The organization should ensure the following :

(a) Documented procedures/work instructions for each activity under study.

(b) Use of approved materials

(c) Use of qualified equipments

(d) The calibration status of measuring devices

(e) The work environment suitability.

(f) The trained manpower

Hence, for production process, the key inputs are Materials, Equipments, Methods, Measuring devices and Manpower.

2.14.2 Validation of Production Process

The organization should validate the documented process and demonstrate that the product manufactured through this established process will be consistent and meet with the established specifications and an additional customers specification as applicable.

The organization should establish the following documents :

(a) Master validation plan document
(b) Validation of facility
(c) Validation of manufacturing process
(d) Equipments cleaning method validation
(e) Drying and blending processes validation
(f) Analytical methods validation
(g) Competency of personnel
(h) Re-validation criteria as applicable

2.14.3 Identification and Traceability

The organization should establish the identification of materials, equipment, and facility as appropriate in all the activities of the manufacturing organization.

The organization should establish the following :

(a) Identification of materials at the input stage, inspection phase and storage. Traceability is an essential requirement. The identification status can be either through appropriate label or status board or location marking.
(b) The identification is an essential requirement because the organization has to use only approved materials in the process.
(c) The suitable identification of equipments is required to establish its suitability, cleaning and operation status.
(d) The identification and calibration status of measuring devices is a requirement to establish its use in the process.
(e) The safety precautions and appropriate re-testing of materials to ensure its suitability over a period of time need to be established.
(f) The handling of materials should be established.

2.14.4 Customer Property

The organization should take proper care of the customer property (contract manufacturing) in identification, verification, protection and storage of materials received from contract giver, as long as these materials are in organization's control. The damaged or lost materials or materials found not suitable for process should be returned to the contract giver and the record should be maintained.

2.14.5 Preservation of Product

This clause pertains to the process of preservation of the finished product from the stage of initial manufacturing operation to the dispatch of the finished product to the customer. This is further extended till the receipt of the finished product by the customer. The organization needs to establish a procedure to describe all the stages from processing to the destiny of the product to the customer.

The procedure should address the following processes.

(a) The input materials
(b) During manufacturing stages
(c) Finished product
(d) Packaging and labeling
(e) Distribution of product
(f) Transportation stage
(g) Receipt of product by the customer.

Each of the process stages include:

(a) Receipt and identification
(b) Storage and handling
(c) Protection during storage
(d) Packaging and distribution.

2.15 Control of Monitoring and Measuring Devices

The organization should establish a procedure/policy for controlling the measuring devices that are being used during various stages of manufacturing. The controlling of devices means to evidence the conformity of measurements.

The organization should establish the procedure to calibrate or verify these measuring devices at defined intervals to ensure their suitability in the manufacturing operations.

The Calibration procedure should include the following :

(a) Calibration procedure, which should define parameters and their acceptance criteria based on the accuracy of the device.
(b) Frequency period for calibration depending on the use of the device.
(c) Calibration should include reference standard and validity of external national standard used in the measurement.

(d) Calibration status identification.

(e) Environmental conditions should be specified if they influence the measurements.

(f) Protection of the measuring devices during their use.

(g) When these measuring devices are found out of calibration, how to validate the previous results.

(h) The measuring devices include computer software.

2.16 Measurement, Analysis and Improvement

2.16.1 General

The organization should demonstrate that the identified processes/activities in the manufacturing operations which are under implementation should cover the phases of installation, monitoring, measurement, analysis of data, and improvements there on over a period of time on continuous basis.

This clause in particular demonstrate the evidence of implementation of Quality Management system, hence should include the following :

(a) To demonstrate conformity and consistency of the product.

(b) Conformity of Quality management System implementation as per the design.

(c) To demonstrate improvements in the business results.

(d) To demonstrate plans to continually improve upon the effectiveness of Quality Management System.

(e) To demonstrate the use of applicable statistical techniques in the analysis of data.

2.16.2 Monitoring and Measurement

Every process which is under implementation of Quality management System needs to be monitored continuously and the measurements made are to be evaluated periodically to ensure effective implementation of the system to yield business results.

Primarily, the monitoring and measurement processes include :

(a) Customer satisfaction.

(b) Internal quality audit.

(c) Manufacturing process.

(d) Quality of the product.

2.16.3 Customer Satisfaction

The key performance indicator on which the entire Quality Management System revolves around is "Customer". This is because "customer" is the purpose of the business.

The organization has to develop a policy to identify, protect, maintain and improve upon the customers to sustain and grow in business.

Generally, customers are divided into two categories.

(a) *Internal customer :* customer within the organization who produces the product at various stages.

(b) *External customer :* customer who uses the finished product outside the organization.

The organization should develop a procedure to monitor and measure the customer satisfaction index, which should include :

(a) Identification of customer
(b) Understanding customer requirements
(c) Performance measurement indicators
(d) Frequency of evaluation
(e) Performance index based on measurements
(f) Identification of new strategies

2.16.4 Internal Audit

The internal audit or self-inspection programme aims at determination of overall performance of the Quality Management System.

The performance of the system need to be evaluated at defined intervals in order to create confidence to the Management that,

(a) Quality Management System conforms to requirements.
(b) Effective implementation and its maintenance.

Thus internal audit results indicate the status of implementation and demonstrate that the system produces desired results and indicates that the system is under control.

The internal audit procedure should include the following :

(a) The audit schedule include annual and periodical.
(b) The audit scope and criteria.
(c) The frequency and duration.
(d) The methodology and check-list.
(e) Selection of auditors.

(f) Recording of observations/non-conformities.
(g) Verification of corrective actions.
(h) Reporting of critical and major non-conformities to the top management.
(i) Review of effectiveness of implementation of corrective actions taken.
(j) Concise summary to top management.

2.16.5 Monitoring and Measurement of Processes

The organization should establish a document titled "product file" which include at least the following :

(a) Facility and work environment status.
(b) Equipments specifications and their operation status.
(c) Technology of the process.
(d) Recording document.
(e) Verification of production documents and records.
(f) Validation document.
(g) Measuring devices calibration status.
(h) Trained manpower.
(i) Analysis of process at defined intervals.

The organization should establish the following :

(a) Process validation document.
(b) Re-validation criteria.
(c) Trend data reports.
(d) Notification of changes to statutory authorities.

2.16.6 Monitoring and Measurement of Product

The organization should establish the following :

(a) Specifications and testing methods for materials.
(b) The measuring devices operation and calibration status.
(c) The methods validations.
(d) The facility and work environment.
(e) Trained and competent manpower.
(f) Use of appropriate reference materials.
(g) Stability data to support expiry dates.
(h) Key quality parameters trend data.

(i) Complaints.
(j) Product recall and return.
(k) Deviations and out of specifications materials handling.
(l) Notification of changes to statutory authorities.

Inorder to address the above issues, organization should establish "Laboratory Manual" document.

2.17 Control of Manufacturing Product

The organization should develop a procedure to address the following :

(a) Product/process criteria
(b) Monitoring criteria
(c) Recording mechanism of non-conformities
(d) Action to be taken to eliminate non-conformity
(e) Re-verification of corrected product
(f) Action to be taken to address non-conformity of product after delivery to customer
(g) Notification of changes to statutory authorities

This process of evaluation is required in the organization primarily to prevent unauthorized/unapproved product entering the manufacturing process and finally to the customer.

2.18 Analysis of Data

The organization should develop a procedure to address the following :

(a) Identification of parameters
(b) Collection of data
(c) Analysis of data
(d) Conclusions

The analysis of data and conclusions drawn based on verification of data will demonstrate the suitability and effective implementation of Quality Management System.

The analysis of data should at least cover the following areas :

(a) Customer satisfaction
(b) Product/process conformance reports
(c) Trend charts for product characteristics and process parameters

(d) Suppliers evaluation data
(e) Internal audit reports
(f) Deviations
(g) Periodic review of Quality Management System

The executive summary can be compiled and documented in a report titled "Annual product Review Report", which should be released at least annually.

2.19 Improvement

2.19.1 Continual Improvement

In order to establish evidence of continual improvement of Quality Management System, the organization should periodically and continually monitor the following :

(a) Quality policy and objectives.
(b) Analysis of data.
(c) Corrective and preventive actions taken especially on critical issues.
(d) Internal audit reports.
(e) Management review reports.

2.19.2 Corrective Action

When non-conformity occurs in the system, the organization shall define a system of identifying non-conformity, the root cause for such non-conformity and action to be initiated to eliminate the non-conformity to prevent recurrence. The corrective action procedure should address the following :

(a) Identification of non-conformity
(b) Investigation of non-conformity (root cause analysis, correction and corrective action)
(c) Action to prevent recurrence of the problem
(d) Verification of implementation of action taken
(e) Periodical review of corrective action taken
(f) Record of results taken.

2.19.3 Preventive Action

The organization should investigate the problems/identified non-conformities, review and categorize as nonpotential and potential non-conformities.

Non-potential non-conformity :

The non-potential non-conformities are those, which do not have a potential impact on the quality of the product.

Potential non-conformity :

The potential non-conformities are those that have a potential impact on the quality and use of the product. The potential non-conformities demand the organization to stop further manufacturing operations till they are corrected.

The organization should establish a procedure to address the following :

(a) Identification of non-conformities.

(b) Review and categorization of non-conformities.

(c) Action to prevent occurrence of potential non-conformity.

(d) Review process of monitoring the preventive actions.

(e) Records.

Summary

The ISO 9000 is a series of international standards on quality management and quality assurance system, which can be adopted by all types of organizations producing and supplying all kinds of goods, services, software etc.,

The ISO 9000 standards also require that a company maintain control of its documented procedures that describe its methods for design, production, inspection, handling, storage and delivery of all materials and products as well as defining the system. This assures continuous employee training and development.

Quality management systems approach :

An approach for developing and implementing a quality management system consists of several steps. For organizations to function effectively, they have to identify and manage numerous interrelated and interacting processes. The systematic identification and management of the processes employed within an organization and particularly the interactions between such processes are referred to as the "Process approach".

The supplier organization should establish, document, implement, monitor and continuously improve the effectiveness of the quality management system (QMS) that should fulfill the requirements of the international QMS as per ISO 9001: 2000.

The supplier Organization should develop Quality Management System documentation based on the process approach concept and should be sound like a pyramid.

Quality manual :

The Quality manual, which is a level-I document of the organisation to include policy statements and should address all the elements / requirements specified in ISO-9001 : 2000 guidance document.

Control of documents :

The Organization should establish a single documented procedure to detail the structure of a procedure and/or work instruction.

The documented procedure should be a key document of the Organization on which the entire documentation structure is based.

Control of records :

Primarily, a record is a document when filled with the data. Record is an evidence of implementation or conformity to the requirements specified in the process. Thus, a record is the proof of implementation status and hence, should not be tampered.

Role of top management within the quality management system :

Through leadership and actions, top management can create an environment where people can involve and achieve a quality management system which can operate effectively. The quality management principles can be used by top management as a tool.

Management commitment :

Top management, which includes proprietor, owner and / or person responsible for business growth, should provide commitment with conviction to develop QMS system and implement and continually improve the effectiveness of implementation through an effective internal audit system.

Customer Focus

Quality policy and Quality objectives :

Quality policy and quality objectives are established to provide a focus to direct the organization. Both determine the desired results and assist the organization to apply its resources to achieve these results. The quality policy provides a framework for establishing and reviewing quality objectives. The quality objectives need to be consistent with the quality policy and the commitment to continual improvement, and their achievement needs to be measurable. The achievement of quality objectives can have a positive impact on product quality, operational effectiveness and financial performance and thus on the satisfaction and confident of interested parties.

Quality objectives :

The Top Management team should frame the quality objectives, which are a means to achieve the Quality Policy.

Responsibility, authority and communication :

Top management should frame and release a document titles "Organization Chart" which should include the reporting hierarchy in the Organization. The responsibilities and authorities of personnel should be documented. The responsibilities of personnel need to be defined explicitly and should be communicated to all personnel within the organization.

Management review :

"Management review" as this term sounds should include the review of activities within the Organization by the Management at defined intervals to understand the current status and assess opportunities to achieve business goals. This is defined as a "process".

Resource management

Provision of resources :

The organization should establish a procedure to define the methodology to provide the necessary resources, which include,

- Technological Resource
- Facility Resource
- Infrastructure resource
- Human Resource
- Business development resource

The required resources need to be identified through Management review process.

Product Realisation :

Planning of product realisation :

The Organization should plan and develop the process for product realisation. The Organization should develop a document, usually referred to as "Quality plan" that should be applies either product based or project based.

Facility	:	Verification and validation report
Equipment	:	Inspection and testing record
Process document	:	Product acceptance record
		Customer satisfaction record

Designs and Development

This phase of study refers to Research and Development function in the organization. This activity can be extended to new product and/or process discovery and/or existing product process modifications or changes as applicable.

Purchasing

Purchasing process :

The organization should ensure the conformity of the materials with the established specifications. The organization should evaluate the implication of these purchased materials on the finished product manufactured by the organization. The quality of the finished product hence depends upon the quality of the input materials supplied either through manufacturers or suppliers. Hence, the need indirectly is on the quality of the suppliers and/or original manufacturers.

Production and service operations :

This requirement/process deals with the various activities that are need to be performed in the manufacturing which cover the following :

(a) Production process and service operations

(b) Validation of applicable processes

(c) Materials identification, storage and trace ability

(d) Customers property/material

(e) Packaging and delivery of the product

(f) Monitoring and measuring devices control and calibration.

Measurement, Analysis and Improvement

General :

The organization should demonstrate that the identified processes/ activities in the manufacturing operations which are under implementation should cover the phases of installation, monitoring, measurement, analysis of data, and improvements there on over a period of time on continuous basis.

This clause in particular demonstrate the evidence of implementation of Quality Management system.

Control of non-conforming product :

The organization should develop a procedure to address the following :

(a) Product/process criteria

(b) Monitoring criteria

(c) Recording mechanism of non-conformities

(d) Action to be taken to eliminate non-conformity

(e) Re-verification of corrected product

(d) Action to be taken to address non-conformity of product after delivery to customer

(e) Notification of changes to statutory authorities

This process of evaluation is essential in the organization primarily to prevent unauthorized/unapproved product entering the manufacturing process and finally to the customer.

Analysis of data :

The organization should develop a procedure to address the following :

(a) Identification of parameters

(b) Collection of data

(c) Analysis of data

(d) Conclusions

Improvement

Continual improvement :

Inorder to establish evidence of continual improvement of Quality Management System, the organization should periodically and continually monitor the following :

(a) Quality policy and objectives

(b) Analysis of data

(c) Corrective and preventive actions taken especially on critical issues

(d) Internal audit reports

(e) Management review reports

Questions

1. Write brief note on evolution of ISO 9000 series standards?
2. What are the different levels of documents to be maintained by an organisation for developing the documentation required in the organisation?
3. What is a document ? What is a record?
4. Define Quality Policy? Frame a typical Quality policy for an Educational university?
5. Define a process? Briefly explain the different activities of a process of executing a commercial order received from a customer?
6. Write a brief note in describing the process of resolving a customer complaint.
7. What are the key items to be included in a management review process?
8. What are the different phases involved from design to commercialization of a new product with specific reference to Quality Management system requirements?
9. Define the term "Validation". Briefly describe the stages and the details to be included to validate on established process.
10. Define the term "Calibration" Briefly describe the requirements and methodology involved to calibrate a temperature gague by own external agency.
11. Define "Customer". How do you measure the customer satisfaction in a service industry?
12. Define the term "Internal Audit". What are key attributes of an Auditor?
13. Define the following terms :
    (a) Correction
    (b) Corrective action
    (c) Preventive action
14. What are the key areas to be considered while analyzing the data in a typical manufacturing organisation?
15. Briefly describe the typical statistical tools required in assessing the performance of a pharmaceutical substance manufacturer.

3

Good Laboratory Practice (GLP)

3.1 Introduction

The term "Good Practice" indicates an established way of doing or performing of an activity in the way that is generally recognized as being the proper one. Today, in this competitive area the "Good Practice" is applicable in every sphere of life starting with "Good Home Practice" and ending with "Good Ethical Practice". The term "Good Laboratory Practice" is distinctly different from others in which, the rules of Good Laboratory Practice is of fundamental importance and necessary in the area of investigation in finding out the safety of chemical products and more so in the field of pharmaceutical manufacturing and testing.

It also describes the recommended practices in judging for "positive" response and to avoid hazardous substances, which affect the environment, and finally human health. In order to prevent or avoid such environmental risks, which might lead to a potential threat to human, and wherever possible, legislation has been introduced worldwide.

Good Laboratory Practice (GLP) in general symbolizes the "good practices" which need to be used in the laboratory, the purpose of which is testing the physical, chemical and microbial testing of materials as applicable and to avoid threat or hazardous to humans.

"Good Laboratory Practices" are a quality system, which establishes accurate documentation covering all aspects of a study and its environment with regard to quality and integrity and reliability of safety data. The GLP have been formulated primarily to promote the quality and validity of test data used for determining the safety of the products. The Quality system of GLP process include the conditions under which Laboratory studies are planned, performed, monitored, and recorded.

3.2 History of GLP

The term "Good Laboratory Practice" was first officially used in the year 1972 in New Zealand Testing Laboratory, where the development and maintenance of Good Laboratory Practice in testing was made mandatory for registration of a "Testing Laboratory"

After the "Thalidomide" disaster the regulatory requirements for "Safety and Testing" of pharmaceuticals were tightened all over the world especially in contract research organizations.

USFDA has first published regulations for GLP in non-clinical laboratory studies in the Federal Legister in the year 1978, the summary of these regulations is to study of quality and integrity of a "product to assure product safety". Like wise, Federal Insecticide, Fungicide and Rodenticide Act which deals with pesticides and their safety and the Toxic Substances Control Act (TSCA) which deals with chemical substances safety, and have separately published GLP regulations by US Environmental Protection Agency (US-EPA) under 40 CFR 160 and 40 CFR 792 respectively in early 80s and subsequently thereon, two regulations have been integrated under 40 CFR 806 by USEPA in the year 1999.

Organization of Economic Cooperation and Development (OECD), which is, an intergovernmental organization with 29 industrialized countries in North America, Europe, Pacific & EU have initiated the task to harmonise these standards in the international trade of chemicals, agrochemicals and pharmaceutical business. The primary purpose of these international standards is to avoid duplicate testing and optimally use monitory and human resource. The expert group on GLP of OECD Council has officially published GLP document in 1981 which states "Data generated in the testing of chemicals in an OECD member country in accordance with OECD test guide lines and principles of Good Laboratory Practice shall be accepted in other member countries for purposes of assessment and other uses relating to the protecting of man and environment".

Subsequently, Netherlands, Switzerland, UK and Japan have formulated their GLP standards. In early 80s European Community has formally adopted OECD guidelines on GLP in their directive 67/18/EEC. In later 80s, the OECD Directorate of Environmental Health and Safety Division had revised OECD principles of GLP in 1997.

The spirit of GLP regulations is to address the various levels in the organization's facility to perform "Safety Studies" and these are mainly regarded as "common sense" approach.

3.3 The Three Basic Issues of GLP are :

3.3.1 To reconstruct and/or do the whole course of safety study for reassurance as needed by the regulatory authority.

3.3.2 To have accountability of GLP study.

3.3.3 To increase GLP awareness among other countries especially in developing countries.

Thus the summary of GLP is to ensure and assure quality and integrity of the test data.

3.4 The Four Quadrants of 'Good Laboratory Practice' are :

3.4.1 The Management

3.4.2 The Quality Assurance

3.4.3 The Study Director

3.4.4 The National Compliance Monitoring Authority

3.4.1 The Management

The organization's management should be in the first place should get convinced that GLP is a good practice to adopt into one's facility voluntarily. After accepting GLP practice, Management should be ultimately responsible for ensuring full compliance throughout the facility. Thirdly, the Management's responsibility is to appoint adequate number of approximately qualified and experienced staff throughout the organization functions and especially on QA function.

3.4.2 The Quality Assurance

The QA functional responsibility involve that the GLP principles appropriate to each area of operation are fully understood to its spirit and observed in the test facility to ensure compliance with these principles. The responsible person, an appointment by Management should have direct access to different levels of Management, especially Top Management level. QA function should be to bringout any deviations from observance of GLP principles in the test facility. The corrective actions taken should be reviewed with the concerned function, and ensure compliance. In essence, QA function should be a bridge between Management and different individual functions.

3.4.3 The Study Director

The focus is on one single responsible person mainly from QA function, appointed by Management, called study director, on whom the whole study depends. The study director key responsibility is to issue that all administrative, scientific and regulatory aspects of the study are fully controlled and ensure that the final report of the study is signed by the study director. The study director should normally be a technical person who will be able to design and approve the study plan, should oversee the study activity while collecting the data, analysis and reporting and should finally draw the conclusions from the study.

3.4.4 National Compliance Monitoring Authority

Like the study Director who is the monitoring agency in the Management site of the test facility, a representative from national monitoring authorities from Government, whose responsibility is to conduct laboratory inspections and audits for compliance. The following are some of the prominent compliance maintenance authorities.

- US Food and Drug Administration, USFDA
- US Environmental Protection Agency, USEPA
- 40 CFR 160 (Federal insecticide, Fungicide and Rodenticide Act)
- 40 CFR 792 (Toxic Substances Control Act)
- 21 CFR, part 58 (USFDA- GLP for non clinical facility)

Applicability

GLP as described above is an inspection / audit by National Regulatory Authority for compliance before issuing license, the authority should verify Quality system, which is a mandatory for its safety testing of materials and the results.

3.5 Responsibilities Matrix

3.5.1 Management

The Management, should provide an optimal environment for conducting GLP compliance of the test facility. It is the responsibility of the Management to provide sufficient number of qualified personnel, appropriate facilities, equipment and materials for timely and proper conduct of the study. It is responsibility of the Management, to ensure that personnel clearly understand the functions they need to perform and where necessary provide training for these functions.

The Management, should appoint study director with appropriate qualifications, training and experience before the study is initiated. In the event of termination of employment of a study director, the Management should replace this position and replacement should be as per the established documented procedure. The study director can appoint principal investigator to act on his behalf in the event of multisite facility study. The Study Director should approve the study plan and should be made available to Quality Assurance personnel. It is the responsibility of the Management that the deviations in the test study are reported by Quality Assurance and are communicated to the Study Director. The corrective actions taken are documented. The Management should ensure that SOPS are established and are being followed as required. The management should ensure that computer systems are suitable for intended purpose, and are validated, operated and maintained in accordance with the principles of GLP.

3.5.2 Study Director

Study Director has the principal responsibility for conduct of the study as per the approved study plan, co-ordinate the activities during the study and for final report preparation and approval.

Study Director should design the study plan and approve, should identify and appoint principal investigator, where required and should approve the test facilities and test site.

Should supervise the activities during the study and ensure that the experimental procedures laid down are followed, samples are collected as per the established sampling plans and observations are recorded to maintain the integrity of the study.

Should ensure that all raw data generated are fully documented and recorded.

Should ensure that computerized systems in use are validated.

Should ensure that study plan, raw data, supporting materials and final report is prepared.

The principal investigator should ensure that delegated phases of the study are conducted in accordance with the applicable GLP.

3.5.3 Study Personnel

The personnel involved in the study team should be knowledgeable, especially in the parts of their involvement in the study, the knowledge include on GLP and SOPS.

The personnel should document any deviations in the study plan and communicate these deviations to study director.

The Personnel are responsible for the quality of the raw data recorded.

The personnel should take utmost precautions to maintain sound health and in the event of any abnormality in health conditions, should report to study director.

3.5.4 The Sponsor

The sponsor should be aware of the concerned regulatory authority requirements. To choose the sponsor, submits the package of non-clinical health and environmental safety studies data to support product registration.

The sponsor should be knowledgeable with the requirements of the GLP principles. The sponsor should evaluate the test facility, facility management and study director, and the scope of the study. The final report should be thoroughly reviewed for compliance with the current GLP principles before the submission of the dossier to the regulatory authority.

3.6 Quality Assurance in GLP

The term 'Quality' has to be viewed to assess an estimate of the reliability of analytical results achieved. The term 'Quality Assurance' must consist of conducting inspections at the test facility to ascertain that all related activities conform to GLP standards. Auditing reports of the study reflects the raw data of the study, Quality Assurance personnel should check the format context of study plans for compliance with the GLP principles. Quality Assurance personnel must acquire the expertise and experience to fulfill their primary responsibilities through training. Apart from this QA personnel must be familiar with company procedures, standards and systems that are being under operation. Quality Assurance personnel need to have good auditing and communication skills.

3.6.1

During the inspections of the study, QA must assure that all the studies are conducted in accordance with the principles of good laboratory practice. Second, the inspections have to be performed frequently to enable QA to judge GLP compliance on continuous basis. The different types of inspections include :

- Facility based inspections
- Study based inspections
- Process based inspections

The different activities that are to be performed in an inspection by QA should include the following but not limited to ;

1. The study Director should approve the study plan.
2. The study plan should be available to QA personnel.
3. The study plan should contain all the information pertaining to the study.
4. The QA personnel should plan for the audit/inspection with the requirements of the GLP principles.
5. The QA personnel should prepare a check-list for the inspection which should cover all the principles of GLP requirements.
6. The QA personnel should prepare a written inspection report and submit to Management and to study Director.
7. The QA should review of the corrective action reports, of the issues included in the report; evaluate the status of compliance and to ensure effectiveness of implementation.
8. The QA personnel should prepare a final report based on the review.
9. Based on the objective of the study, review of data and reports, the QA should conclude and summarize in the final QA statement or certificate of compliance.

3.6.2 GLP-Implementation and Organisation

OECD countries have implemented GLP after obtaining the necessary legislative and administrative support. They have introduced GLP compliance monitoring by periodic inspection of laboratories and auditing of studies through a National GLP Compliance Programme under the aegis of a National GLP Monitoring Authority with the responsibility of monitoring the GLP compliance of laboratories. Under this programme on behalf of the monitoring authority an inspector conducts an on-site examination of test facility's procedures and practices to assess the degree of compliance.

During the inspection, the management structure and operational procedures of the laboratory are examined, key technical personnel are interviewed, and the quality and integrity of data generated by the facility are assessed by a comparison of data and associated records with the interim or final report. This reveals whether testing is carried out in accordance with the protocol and the standard operating procedures and whether the quality assurance programme is adequate to assure the management that the studies are conducted in accordance with the GLP principles.

3.6.3 Organisation of a GLP Monitoring Unit

This comprises a Director under whose guidance trained inspectors operate.

The inspectors should be scientifically and academically qualified and should have practical experience in Toxicological/Analytical Chemistry. They should have knowledge of chemical and pharmaceutical industries and must be familiar with GLP requirements, Compliance Standards and regulations in other countries.

The inspectors are responsible for maintenance of confidentiality. They have access to highly confidential and commercially valuable information. The information should be protected under the provisions of the Official Secrets Act. All information acquired is classified as "Commercial in Confidence".

The inspectors carry a means of their identification. The inspected laboratory should posses compliance statements, summary of inspection reports, special study audits, etc. These could, if necessary, be made available to regulatory authorities to emphasise the high quality and validity of the data submitted.

3.6.4 GLP Status in INDIA

In India, Laboratories which conduct studies in accordance with GLP Principles are only very few though some may claim to do so. Without the presence of any GLP Compliance Monitoring Authority, any such claim cannot be verified. Assurance of safety/analytical standards to international specification by GLP certified laboratories would help in participation in international competition among various consumer products, drugs, pesticides, industrial chemicals in both the domestic and export markets. There is, therefore, an urgent need to increase the awareness about GLP and initiate actions to facilitate introduction of GLP in all Indian Laboratories. Currently none of the Indian Government departments have a GLP certification scheme.

3.7 Calibration and Testing (General Requirements for Competent Calibration and Testing Lab)

3.7.1 Introduction

Many countries have adopted ISO/IEC Guide 25 as the basis both for establishing quality systems in laboratories and for recognizing their competence, e.g. by accreditation. In recent years there have been many developments in the field of quality assurance, which have led to new and improved guides and standards; it was recognized that there was a need to revise ISO/IEC Guide 25 to reflect these changes.

In this revision of the Guide, attention is paid to the activities of both calibration and testing laboratories and account is taken of other requirements for laboratory competence such as those laid down in the OECD Code of Good Laboratory Practice IGLP and the ISO 9000 series of quality assurance standards.

This Guide should provide a mechanism for promoting confidence in calibration and testing laboratories that can show that they operate in accordance with its requirements.

Acceptance of calibration and test results between countries will facilitate the removal of non-tariff barriers to trade.

The use of this Guide will facilitate cooperation between laboratories and other bodies to assist in the exchange of information and experience, and in the harmonization of standards and procedures.

This Guide is specific to calibration laboratories and testing laboratories. Laboratories meeting the requirements of this Guide comply, for calibration and testing activities, with the relevant requirements of the ISO 9000 series of standards, including those of the model described in ISO 9002 when they are acting as suppliers producing calibration and test results.

3.7.2 Scope

This Guide sets out the general requirements in accordance with which a laboratory has to demonstrate that it operates, if it is to be recognized as competent to carry out specific calibrations objects.

This Guide is for use by calibration and testing laboratories in the development and implementation of their quality systems. It may also be used by accreditation bodies, certification bodies and others concerned with the competence of laboratories.

3.7.3 References

ISO 8402 : 1986. Quality Vocabulary

ISO 9000 : 1987. Quality management and quality assurance standards – Guidelines for selection and use.

ISO 9001 : 1987. Quality systems Model for quality assurance in design/ development, production, installation and servicing.

ISO 9002 : 1987. Quality systems-Model for quality assurance in production and installation.

ISO 9003 : 1987. Quality systems Model for quality assurance in final inspection and test.

ISO 9004 : 1987. Quality management and quality system elements-Guidelines.

ISO/IEC Guide 2 : 1986. General terms and their definitions concerning standardization and related activities.

3.7.4 Definitions

The relevant definitions from ISO/IEC Guide 2. ISO 8402 and the International vocabulary of basic and general terms in metrology are applicable, the most relevant being quoted below together with further definitions applicable for the purposes of this Guide.

Laboratory : Body that calibrates and/or tests.

Notes :

1. In cases where a laboratory forms part of an organization that carries out other activities besides calibration and testing, the term "Laboratory" refers only to those parts of that organization that are involved in the calibration and testing process.
2. As used herein, the term "laboratory" refers to a body that carries out calibration or testing.
   - At or from a permanent location.
   - At or from a temporary facility, or
   - In or from a mobile facility.

   Testing laboratory: Laboratory that performs tests.

   [ISO/IEC Guide 2-12.4]

   Calibration laboratory : Laboratory that performs calibration.

Calibration : The set of operations, which establish, under specified conditions, the relationship between values indicated by a measuring instrument or measuring system, or values represented by a material measurement, and the corresponding values of the measured.

Notes :

1. The result of a calibration permits the estimation of errors of location of the measuring instrument, measuring system or material measure or the assignment of values to marks on arbitrary scales.
2. A calibration may also determine other meterology properties.
3. The result of a calibration may be recorded in a document some time called calibration certificate or a calibration report.
4. The result of a calibration is sometimes expressed as a calibration factor or as a series of calibration factors in the from of a calibration.

Test : A technical operation that consists of the determination of one or more characteristics or performance of a given produce material equipment, organism, physical phenomenon, process or service according to a specific procedure.

Note : The result of a test is normally recorded in a document sometimes called a test report or a test certificate.

Calibration method : Defined technical procedure for conforming a calibration.

Test method : Defined technical procedure for performing a test.

Verification: confirmation by examination and provision of evidence that specified requirements have been met.

Note : In connection with the management of measuring equipment, verification provides a means for checking that the deviations between values of a measured quantity are consistently smaller than the maximum allowable error defined in a standard, regulation or specification peculiar to the management of the measuring equipment.

The result of verification leads to a decision either to restore to service, or to perform adjustments, or to repair or to downgrade or to declare obsolete. In all cases it is required that a written trace of the verification performed be kept on the measuring instrument's individual record.

Quality system : The organizational structure, responsibilities, procedures, processes and resources for implementing quality management.

Quality manual : A document stating the quality policy, quality system and quality practices of an organization.

Note : The quality manual may call up other documentation relating to the laboratory quality arrangements.

Reference standard : A standard generally of the highest meteorological quality available at a given location from which measurements are made.

Reference material : A material or substance one or more properties of which are sufficiently well established to be used for the calibration of an apparatus, the assessment of a measurement method, or for assigning values to materials.

Certified reference material (CRM) : A reference material one or more of whose property values are by a technically valid procedure accompanied by traceability certificate or other documentation which is issued by a certifying body.

Traceability : The property issued by where by it can be related to appropriate generally international or national standards, through an uncertain of comparisons.

Proficiency testing : determination to the library calibration or sting performance by means of necessary comparisons.

Requirement : A translation of the needs into a set of individual quantified or descriptive specifications for the characteristics of an entity in order to enable its realization and examination.

3.8 Organization and Management

The laboratory shall be legally identifiable. It shall be organized and shall operate in such a way that its permanent, temporary and mobile facilities meet, the requirements of this Guide.

3.9 Quality System, Audit and Review

The laboratory shall establish and maintain a quality system appropriate to the type, range and volume of calibration and testing activities it undertakes. The elements of this system shall be documented. The quality documentation shall be available for use by the laboratory personnel. The laboratory shall define and document its policies and objectives and its commitment to Good laboratory practice and quality of calibration or testing services. The laboratory management shall ensure that these policies and objectives are documented in a quality manual and communicated to, understood, and implemented by all laboratory personnel concerned. The quality manual shall be maintained current under the responsibility of the quality manager.

3.10 Personnel

The testing laboratory shall have sufficient personnel, having the necessary education, training, technical knowledge and experience for their assigned functions.

The testing laboratory shall ensure that the training of its personnel up to date.

Records on the relevant qualifications, training, skills and experience of the technical personnel shall be maintained by the laboratory.

3.11 Accommodation and Environment

Laboratory accommodation, calibration and test areas, energy sources, lighting, heating and ventilation shall be such as to facilitate proper performance of calibrations or tests.

The environment in which these activities are undertaken shall not invalidate the results or adversely affect the required accuracy of measurement. Particular care shall be taken when such activities are undertaken at sites other than the permanent laboratory premises.

The laboratory shall provide facilities for the effective monitoring control and recording of environmental conditions as appropriate. Due attention shall be paid, for example to biological sterility, dust, electromagnetic interference, humidity, mains voltage, temperature, and sound and vibration levels, as appropriate to the calibrations or tests concerned.

There shall be a distinct separation between neighbouring areas when the activities therein are incompatible.

Access to and use of all areas affecting the quality of these activities shall be defined and controlled.

Accurate measures shall be taken to ensure good housekeeping in the laboratory.

Note : It is the laboratory responsibility to comply with the relevant health and safety requirements.

3.12 Equipment and Reference Materials

The laboratory shall be furnished with all items and equipments including reference materials required for the source performance of calibrations and tests. In these cases where the laboratory needs to use equipment outside its preview it shall ensure that the relevant requirements of this Guide are met.

All equipment shall be properly maintained. Maintenance procedures shall be documented. Any item of the equipment which has been suspected to overating or misnaming or which gives suspect results, or has been govern by verification or otherwise to be defective shall be taken out of service and wherever possible stored at a specific place until it has been repaired and show calibration certification or test to perform satisfactorily. The organisation shall examine the effect of this on previous calibration or test results.

Each Item of equipment including reference materials shall, when appropriate, be labeled or marked or otherwise certified to indicate its calibration status.

Records shall be maintained of each item of equipment and the records shall include,

(a) The name of the item of equipment.

(b) The manufacturer's name, type certification and serial number or other unique identification.

(c) Date received and date placed in service.

(d) Current location, where appropriate.

(e) Condition when received.

(f) Copy of the manufacturer's instructions, where available.

(g) Dates and results of calibrations and/or verifications and date of next calibration and/or verification.

(h) Details of maintenance carried out to date and planned for the future.

(i) History of any damage, malfunction, modification or repair.

3.13 Measurement Traceability and Calibration

All measuring and testing equipment having an effect on the accuracy or validity of calibrations or tests shall be calibrated and or verified before being put into service. The laboratory shall have an established programme for the calibration and verification of its measuring and test equipment.

The overall Programme of calibration and or verification and validation of equipment shall be designed and operated so as to ensure that wherever applicable, measurements made by the laboratory are traceable to national standards of measurement where available. Calibration certificates shall wherever applicable indicate the traceability to national standards of measurement and shall provide the measurement results and associated uncertainty of measurement and or a statement of committment with an identified meteorological specification.

Where traceability to national standards of measurement is not applicable, the laboratory shall provide satisfactory evidence of correlation of results, for example by participation in a Programme of inter-laboratory comparisons testing.

Reference standards of measurement held by the laboratory shall be used for calibration only and for no other purpose, unless it can be demonstrated that their performance as reference standards has not been invalidated.

Reference standards of measurement shall be calibrated by a body that can provide traceability to a national standard of measurement. There shall be a Programme of calibration and verification of reference standards.

Where relevant, reference standards and measuring and testing equipments shall be subjected to in-service sneaks certified validations certifications.

Reference materials shall where possible to be traceable to national or international standards of measurement or to national or international standard reference materials.

3.14 Calibration and Test Methods

The laboratory shall have documented instructions on the use and operation of all relevant equipment, on the handling and preparation of items and for calibration and/or testing. All instructions, standards, manuals and reference data relevant to the work in the laboratory shall be maintained up-to-date and be readily available to the staff.

The laboratory shall use appropriate methods and procedures for all calibrations and tests and related activities within its responsibility (including sampling, handling, transport and storage, preparation of items, estimation of uncertain of measurement and analysis of calibration and/or test data). They shall be consistent with the accuracy required and with any standard specifications relevant to the calibrations of tests concerned.

Where methods are not specified, the laboratory shall, wherever possible, select methods that have been published in international or national standards, those published by reputable technical organizations or in relevant scientific texts or journals.

Where it is necessary to employ methods that have not been established as standard, these shall be subject to agreement with the client, be fully documented and validated and be available to the client and other recipients.

Where sampling is carried out as part of the test method, the laboratory shall use documented procedures and appropriate statistical techniques to select samples.

Calculations and data transfers shall be subject to appropriate checks.

Where computers or automated equipments are used for the capture, processing, manipulation, recording, reporting, storage or retrieval of calibration or test data, the actual use shall ensure that:

(a) The requirements of this Guide are complied with
(b) Computer software is documented and accurate for use;
(c) Procedures are established and implemented for protecting the integrity of data, such procedures shall include but not be limited to integrity of data entry or capture, data storage, data transmission and data processing.
(d) Computer and automatic equipment's procedures for the maintainance to ensure proper functioning and provided with the environmental and operational conditions as necessary.
(e) It establishes all elements appropriate for the maintenance of security of data including the prevention of unauthorized access to and the unauthorized amendment of computer records.

Documented procedures shall exist for the purchase, reception and storage of consumable materials used for the technical operations of the laboratory.

3.15 Handling of Calibration and Test Items

The laboratory shall have a documented system for uniquely identifying the items to be calibrated or tested, to ensure that there can be no confusion regarding the identity of such items at any time.

Upon receipt, the condition of the calibration or test including any abnormalities or departures from standard condition as prescribed in the relevant calibration or test method, shall be recorded. Where there is any doubt as to the suitability for calibration or test, where the item does not conform to the type of description provided, or where the calibration or test regard is not fully specified, the laboratory shall consult for further instructions before proceeding. The laboratory shall establish whether the item has received all necessary preparation, or whether the client requires preparation to be undertaken or arranged by the laboratory.

The laboratory shall have documented procedures and appropriate facilities to avoid deterioration or damage to the calibration or test item, during storage, handling, preparation, and calibration or test and relevant instructions provided with the item shall be followed. Where items have to be stored or conditioned under specific environmental conditions, these conditions shall be maintained, monitored and recorded where necessary. Where a calibration or test item or portion of an item is to be held secure for example for reasons of record, safety of value or to enable check calibrations or tests to be performed later, the laboratory shall have storage and security arrangements that protect the condition and integrity of the secure items or portions concerned.

Above laboratory shall have documented procedures for the readapt detention or safe disposal of calibration or test items, including all provisions necessary to protect the integrity of the laboratory.

3.15.1 Records

The laboratory shall maintain records system to suit its particular circumstances and comply with any applicable regulations. It shall retain on record all original observations, calculations and derived data calibration records and a copy of the calibration certificate, test certificate or test report for an appropriate period. The records for each calibration and test shall contain sufficient information to permit their repetition the sampling, preparation, calibration or testing.

All records pertaining to calibration and test equipment, certificates and reports shall be safely stored, held secure and in confidence to the client.

3.15.2 Certificates and Reports

The results of each calibration test, or series of calibrations or tests carried out by the laboratory shall be reported accurately, clearly, unambiguously and objectively, in accordance with any instructions in the calibration or test methods. The results should normally be reported in a calibration certificate, test report or test certificate and should include all the information necessary for the interpretation of the calibration or test results and all information required by the method used.

Each certificate or report shall include at least the following information :

(a) a title e.g. "Calibration Certificate", "Test Report" or "Test Certificate".

(b) Name and address of laboratory, and location where the calibration or test was carried out if different from the address of the laboratory

(c) Unique identification of the certificate or report (such as serial number) and of each page, and the total number of pages.

(d) Name and address of client, where appropriate.

(e) Description and unambiguous identification of the item calibrated or tested.

(f) Characterization and condition of the calibration or test item.

(g) Care of receipt of calibration or test item and date (s) of performance of calibration of test, where appropriate;

(h) Identification of the calibration or test method used or unambiguous description of any non-standard method used:

(i) Reference to sampling procedure, where relevant;

(j) Any deviations from additions to or exclude one from the calibration or test method, and any other information relevant to a specific calibration or test such as environmental conditions.

(k) Measurements examinations and derived results supported by tables, graphs, sketches and photographs as appropriate and any failures identified.

(l) A statement of the estimated uncertainty of the calibration or test result where relevant.

(m) A signature and title, or an equivalent certification of the person's accepting responsibility for the content of the certificate or report however produced, and date of issue.

(n) Where relevant a statement to the effect that the results relate only to the items calibrated or tested.

(o) A statement that the certificate shall not be the laboratory

Where the certificate or report contains results of calibrations or tests performed by sub-contractors, these results shall be clearly identified.

Particular care and attention shall be paid to the arrangement of the certificate or report, especially with regard to presentation of the calibration or test data and ease of assimilation by the reader. The format shall be carefully and specifically designed for each type of calibration or test carried out, but the headings shall be standardized as far as possible.

Material amendments to a calibration certificate, test report or test certificate after issue shall be made only in the form of a further document, or data transfer including the statement "Supplement to Calibration Certificate or Test Report or Test Certificate, serial number [or as otherwise identified]", or equivalent form of warding. Such amendments shall meet all the relevant requirements of clause 12 of this Guide.

The laboratory shall notify clients promptly in writing, of any event such as the identification of defective measuring or test equipment that casts doubt on the validity of results given in any calibration certificate, test report or test certificate and amendment to a report or certificate.

The laboratory shall ensure that where clients require transmission of calibration or test results by telephone, telex, facsimile or other electronic or electromagnetic means, staff will follow documented procedures that ensure that the requirements of this Guide are met and that confidentiality is preserved.

Where a laboratory sub-contracts any part of the calibration or testing, this work shall be placed with a laboratory complying with these requirements. The laboratory shall ensure and be able to demonstrate that its sub-contractor is competent to perform the activities in question and complies with the same criteria of competence as the laboratory in respect of the work being sub-contracted. The laboratory shall advise the client in writing of its intention to sub-contract any calibration of the testing to another party.

The laboratory shall record and retain details of its investigation of the competence and compliance or its subcontractors and maintain a register of all sub-contracting.

3.15.3 Outside Support Services and Supplies

Where the laboratory procures outside services and supplies, other than those referred to this Guide, in support of calibrations or tests, the laboratory shall use only these outside support services and supplies that are of adequate quality to sustain confidence in the laboratory's calibrations or tests.

Where no independent assurance of the quality of outside support services or supplies is available, the laboratory shall have procedures to ensure that purchased equipment, materials and services comply with specified requirements. The laboratory should wherever possible, ensure that purchased equipment and consumable materials are not used until they have been inspected, calibrated or otherwise verified as complying with any standard specifications relevant to the calibrations or tests concerned.

3.15.4 Complaints

The laboratory shall have documented policy and procedures for the resolution of complaints received from clients or other parties about the laboratory's activities. A record shall be maintained of all complaints and of the actions taken by the laboratory.

Where a complaint, or any other circumstance raises doubt concerning the laboratory's compliance with the laboratory's policies or procedures, or with the requirements of this Guide or otherwise concerning the quality of the laboratory's calibrations or tests the laboratory shall ensure that those areas of activity and responsibility involved are promptly audited in accordance with this Guide.

Summary

Good Laboratory Practice (GLP) in general symbolizes the "good practices" need to be used in the laboratory, the purpose of which is testing the physical, chemical and microbial testing of materials as applicable and to avoid threat or hazardous to humans.

"Good Laboratory Practices" are a quality system, which establishes accurate documentation covering all aspects of a study and its environment with regard to quality and integrity and reliability of safety data. The GLP have been formulated primarily to promote the quality and validity of test data used for determining the safety of the products. The Quality system of GLP process include the conditions under which Laboratory studies are planned, performed, monitored, and recorded.

History of GLP

The term "Good Laboratory Practice" was first officially used in the year 1972 in New Zealand Testing Laboratory, where the development and maintenance of Good Laboratory Practice in testing was made mandatory for registration of a "Testing Laboratory"

After the "Thalidomide" disaster the regulatory requirements for "Safety and Testing" of pharmaceuticals were tightened all over the world especially in contract research organizations.

USFDA has first published regulations for GLP in non-clinical laboratory studies in the Federal Legister in the year 1978 the summary of these regulations is study of quality and integrity of a "product to assure product safety". Like wise, Federal Insecticide, Fungicide and Rodenticide Act which deals with pesticides and their safety and the Toxic Substances Control Act (TSCA) which deals with chemical substances safety have separately published GLP regulations by US Environmental Protection Agency (US-EPA) under 40 CFR 160 and 40 CFR 792 respectively in early 80s and subsequently thereon, two regulations have been integrated under 40 CFR 806 by USEPA in the year 1999.

Organization of Economic Cooperation and Development (OECD), which is, an intergovernmental organization with 29 industrialized countries in North America, Europe, Pacific & EU have initiated the task to harmonise these standards in the international trade of chemicals, agrochemicals and pharmaceutical business. The primary purpose of these international standards is to avoid duplicate testing and optimally use monitory and human resource. The expert group on GLP of OECD Council has officially published GLP document in 1981 which states "Data generated in the testing of chemicals in an OECD member country in accordance with OECD test guide lines and principles of Good Laboratory Practice shall be accepted in other member countries for purposes of assessment and other uses relating to the protecting of man and environment".

Subsequently, Netherlands, Switzerland, UK and Japan have formulated their GLP standards. In early 80s European Community has formally adopted OECD guidelines on GLP in their directive 67/18/EEC. In later 80s, the OECD Directorate of Environmental Health and Safety Division had revised OECD principles of GLP in 1997.

The spirit of GLP regulations is to address the various organizations levels of a facility to perform "Safety Studies" and which are mainly regarded as "common sense" approach.

The three basic issues of GLP are :

- To reconstruct and/or do the whole course of safety study for reassurance as needed by the regulatory authority.
- To have accountability of GLP study.
- To increase GLP awareness among other countries especially in developing countries.
- Thus, the summary of GLP is to ensure and assure quality and integrity of the test data.

The four quadrants of 'Good Laboratory Practice' are

- The Management
- The Quality Assurance
- The Study Director
- The National Compliance Monitoring Authority

GLP-Implementation and organisation

OECD countries have implemented GLP after obtaining the necessary legislative and administrative support. They have introduced GLP compliance monitoring by periodic inspection of laboratories and auditing of studies through a National GLP Compliance Programme under the aegis of a National GLP Monitoring Authority with the responsibility of monitoring the GLP compliance of laboratories.

During the inspection, the management structure and operational procedures of the laboratory are examined, key technical personnel are interviewed, and the quality and integrity of data generated by the facility are assessed by a comparison of data and associated records with the interim or final report.

Calibration and testing (general requirements for competent calibration and testing lab).

Many countries have adopted ISO/IEC Guide 25 as the basis both for establishing quality systems in laboratories and for recognizing their competence, e.g. by accreditation.

Questions

1. Write down brief historical aspects and evolution of GLP.
2. What are key issues to be considered in implementing GLP in a service-testing Laboratory?
3. What are the four pillions of GLP? Discuss the responsibilities under each item.
4. What is the role of "Quality assurance" in implementing GLP in a pharmaceutical manufacturing industry?
5. Frame the sequential steps required to implement GLP in a pharmaceutical industry Quality Control Laboratory and write down the model.
6. Discuss the general requirements for a competent calibration and testing labs as per ISO/ IEC guide 25 and OECD guide of GLP and ISO respectively?

4

Methods of Analytical Quality Assurance (AQA)

4.1 Introduction

The task of the analyst is to determine the quality of each analytical process he or she uses, and to improve, guarantee, and document it if necessary, so that the achieved quality is maintained at any point during routine analysis. Only then is an analytical process considered reliable.

The objective of analytical work is the achievement of reliable analytical results of a defined quality. Quality characteristics of analytical processes are therefore:

- ***Specificity :*** the ability of an analytical process to register only the desired analyte, while other components or characteristics present in the sample (known as the matrix) do not influence the result.
- ***Sensitivity :*** the change in measured value per change in analyte.
- ***Accuracy :*** in the sense of both trueness (lack of systematic errors) and precision (measurement of differences between results, as obtained by repeated use of an established analytical process on the same sample. Imprecision is caused by random errors).

4.2 Selection of Methods of Chemical Analysis and Sampling

Analytical results are produced in both great number and at great cost, with varying objectives (Table 4.1).

Several subcategories of analytical science are regulated by law, which determines the type and frequency of the analyses performed. Examples of such areas are:

- *Medicine* : epidemic control laws
- *Pharmacy* : drug purity laws
- *Production of materials* : chemical regulations
- *Environmental protection* : drinking water standards, wastewater discharge standards, air emissions standards, etc.

The tasks required of analytical chemistry may generally be seen as the determination of the answer to one of the following five basic questions :

1. Is a substance present in a given sample or not?
2. In which range of concentration is the substance in question present?
3. Is the concentration below appropriate threshold levels?
4. Has a threshold level been exceeded?
5. In what concentration (plus or minus statistical error) is the substance in question present in the sample?

These different questions necessitate varying requirements in the quality of the analytical procedure being used.

4.3 General Differentiation of Analytical Processes

Analytical processes may be categorized into six groups (Table 4.1) based on the objective, the effort required, and the required degree of information to be provided by the results.

Table 4.1 Purposes and uses of analyses

Analytical purpose	Special requirements of analytical process	Examples
1. Detection of harmful Agents, screening	high degree of specificity low limit of detection rapid execution economical	preventive medical examinations (e.g. blood sugar test sticks) toxicology and forensic medicine : identification of poisons and drugs toxin identification and cause determinations in environmental incidents
2. Decision making	high degree of specificity high degree of accuracy	proof in criminology medical diagnostics evaluation of toxic emissions from facilities (threshold limits) determination of fees and penalties (e.g. waste water emissions, solid waste disposal, atmospheric emissions) quality control testing raw material upon receipt from suppliers
3. Ensuring the Protection of people And the environment	high degree of specificity high degree of accuracy	warning systems (e.g. gas detection systems) foodstuff inspections quality control of pharmaceuticals, chemicals, fuels and other materials analyses related to the licensing of
4. Evaluation of process Results	high degree of specificity high degree of accuracy	new or modified technical installations environmental clean-up evaluation of medical therapies
5. Monitoring, process Supervision and Process regulation	high degree of specificity high degree of accuracy rapid execution	process supervision of foodstuff, pharmaceutical, chemical and material production emissions monitoring of environmentally relevant facilities progress control of long term medical therapies
6. General information	high degree of specificity high degree of accuracy rapid execution	basic research in all fields preparation of environmental data bases

4.4 Quality of Analytical Processes and Results

The appropriate analytical process for obtaining the answer to a specific question must not always be the scientifically "best" procedure (Table 4.2). However, it is important that the results of an analysis, obtained through adherence to legal regulations, should if necessary be defensible in court, or in other words legally binding.

Table 4.2 Precision requirements of analytical procedures as related to the analytical problem

Question	Quality required of an analytical process
Is a substance present or not?	Yes/no decision; a sufficiently sensitive orientation test is applicable.
In which range of concentration is the substance is present?	an orientation test indicating a corresponding gradation of concentration regions is applicable.
Does the concentration lie far below A verifiable threshold limit?	A highly precise analytical result is nor necessary; orientation tests and field methods are applicable.
Has a threshold limit been	A highly accurate (meaning both exceeded? precision and trueness) analytical result is required, i.e. only reference procedures and if available comparable laboratory procedures are applicable.
In what concentration, and confidence interval, is the substance in question present in the sample? And standard	A highly accurate (meaning both precision trueness) analytical result is required. If the analytical result is legally binding, only standard methods or comparable laboratory procedures are acceptable. Otherwise, other analytical procedures whose reliability has been proven are applicable.

4.5 Statistical Methods for Analytical Procedure

4.5.1

Statistical methods are used for planning, interpretation and assessment of the data generated by analytical method. The following are the terms used in statistical analysis of analytical data.

4.5.2 Reliability

Quality under set application conditions during or after a set time period.

4.5.3 Measurement Principles

Characteristic physical (Properties, which are used for measurement e.g. photometry).

4.5.4 Measurement Methods

Practical application of measurement principles are :

(a) ***Direct :*** Obtaining measured values by immediate comparison with a reference quantity (e.g. volume measurements).

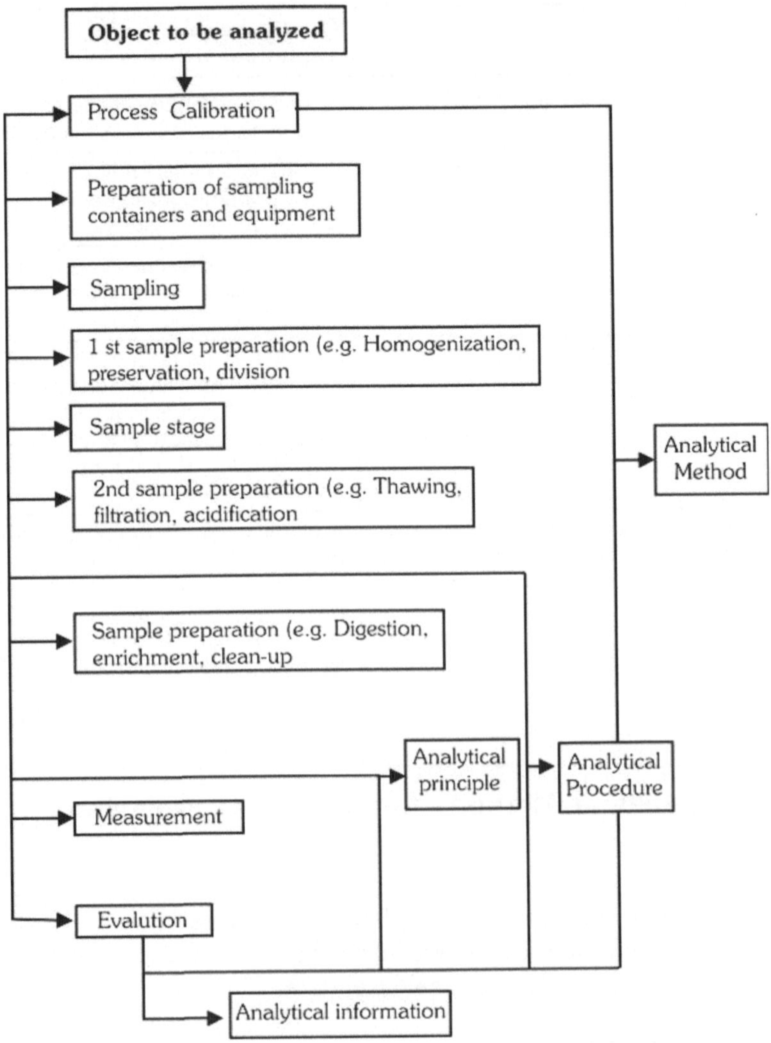

Figure 4.1 Scheme for the terms analytical.

(b) ***Indirect :*** reduction of measured values to different physical quantities (i.e. operational parameters)

4.5.5 Analytical Principle

Refers only to the measurement and the evaluation of measured values (see Scheme).

4.5.6 Analytical Procedure

Refers only to the determination of a defined substance and the evaluation of measured values (see Scheme).

4.5.7 Analytical Method

An analytical process is a combination of processes like preparation (object dependent) sample techniques (sample taking, sample preparation) principle of analytical procedure and analytical method which is shown schematically in Fig. 4.1.

4.5.8 Standard Methods

A standard method is an acknowledged analytical method according to an international or national standard or guideline or to a given legal statute,

Synonyms for standard methods are :

(a) Arbitration methods

(b) Reference methods

4.5.8.1 Standard methods

Which may be national standard procedures, or international (e.g. ASTM, ISO, ECCLES, CEN, IUPAC, etc) guidelines and standards, or procedures described by legal regulations. Standard methods represent the accepted latest state of engineering; their use may be prescribed and/or obligatory within a framework of regulations and guidelines.

4.5.8.2 Comparable laboratory procedures

Quantitative analytical processes which vary in procedure from standard methods, but whose equivalence is verified using standard methods.

4.5.8.3

Other quantitative analytical procedures which have various uses and objectives in the laboratory outside of governmentally regulated areas. These also include the latest analytical procedures for which standards have not yet been established.

4.5.8.4 Field methods

Analytical process which can be performed outside the laboratory. With the aid of objective measurement methods, field methods can bring quantitative or semi-quantitative results depending on previous handling of the sample and quality assurance procedures.

4.5.8.5

Orientation tests assess subjectively; they can qualitatively prove the presence of a certain substance and allow a concentration estimate to be made which is accurate to within one order of magnitude.

4.5.9 True Value

Real (theoretical) characteristic value under conditions prevailing during the analysis.

Note : The true value is often an ideal value because it can only be determined if all errors in the results could be avoided, or is a result of theoretical considerations.

4.5.10 Conventional True Value

A value for the sake of comparison, whose deviation from the true value is considered to be negligible for comparative purposes.

> ***Note 1 :*** The conventional true value is an approximation for the true value. It can be obtained from international, national or usage norms, from reference materials or standard methods (e. g. on the basis of specially organized experiments).
>
> ***Note 2 :*** There are several terms, which are used as synonyms of "conventional true value". Examples are "expected value" and "target value". These terms are ambiguous and should be avoided.

4.5.11 Expected Value

The mean experimental result obtained using a continuously repeated experimental process under established conditions.

4.5.12 Actual value

An analytical result obtained momentarily, generally differentiated from the "expected value" (conventional true value) by the presence of systematic and/or coincidental error.

4.5.13 Accuracy

Accuracy is a qualitative term for the extent of the approximation of analytical results to the reference value, which may be either the true, real or expected value depending on definition or agreement.

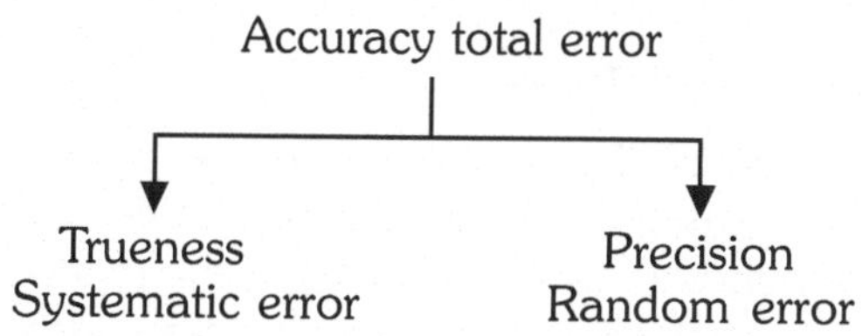

Accuracy is therefore a generic term for precision and trueness.

The determining factor for the overall error is the largest individual error.

The random error may be decreased by a factor $\sqrt{N}$ by repeating the analyses N times.

Systematic error may only be eliminated by the elimination of its cause.

4.5.14 Precision

Precision is a qualitative term for the extent of the mutual approximation of analytical results independent from one another by repeated use of a set analytical process under defined conditions-

The conditions under which analytical results are obtained must be reported exactly, One should notice the distinction between repeatability and reproducibility.

4.5.15 Repeatability, Within Run (or Batch) Precision

Repeatability is a qualitative term for the extent of reciprocal approximation of analytical results under repeat conditions. The terms "precision under repeat conditions" and/or "Serial Precision" may also be used.

Repeat conditions: Conditions for obtaining independent analytical results consisting of the repeated use of a set analytical process or method on the same object (same material, same sample) by the same observer in small time intervals (immediately following each other) with the same equipment (as well as identical supplies and other materials) in the same place (same laboratory).

4.5.16 Reproducibility

Reproducibility is a qualitative term for the extent of reciprocal approximation of analytical results under comparable conditions. The terms "precision under comparable conditions" and/or "precision from lab to lab" are sometimes used in everyday speech.

4.5.17 Analytical Specificity

Analytical specificity is the ability of an experimental process to register only analyte, whereby other components or characteristics present in the sample do not influence the analytical result.

4.5.18 Analytical Sensitivity

Sensitivity describes the ability of an experimental method to differentiate between related values (e.g. concentrations). It indicates to which degree a value changes depending upon the signal of the measuring system and can be quantified using the slope of the calibration curve.

4.5.19 Validation

Validation is the total testing procedure if an analytical method is free of-random and systematic errors, not only within calibration but also and especially free of interferences when analyzing real samples.

National regulations may establish official validation for special measurement instruments, consisting of testing done by the appropriate authorities carried out according to regulations. A validation seal may also be affixed.

4.5.20 Calibration

The calibration of a system is the determination and establishment of a functional relationship between a numerical or measurable quantity and a concentration to be determined (activity, frequency, etc.) from data, which are generally subject to random errors.

4.5.21 Adjustment

Adjustment is setting or aligning a measuring instrument so that measurement errors are kept as small as possible or that the total measurement error does not exceed the limits of error.

4.5.22 Level of Significance P

The level of significance P denotes the relative safety of a "statistical decision".

4.5.23 Bulk Sample

A bulk sample is one taken on the spot, whose content is to be determined quantitatively, the analytical result therefore represents an approximation of the true value.

4.5.24 Analytical Sample

An analytical sample is a sample which is obtained from the bulk -sample after a work-up (e.g. disintegration, extraction, etc.) and, if necessary, dilution (or concentration) and which will be used for the actual measuring process. An analytical sample is therefore identical with a bulk sample if the original sample may be used directly in the measuring process without work-up and dilution (or concentration).

4.5.25 Measurement Sample

A measurement sample is a sample whose content of analyte may be measured directly. A measurement sample is normally obtained from an analytical sample by the addition of a series of reagents. Measurement samples and analytical samples are therefore identical when no reagents are added to the analytical sample.

4.5.26 Mean t-test

A test of the statistical difference between two means ($\overline{x}_1$, $\overline{x}_2$) obtained from two independent series of analyses (normal distribution assumed or required). A testing value TV is calculated and compared with the threshold value t from the t-Table :

$$TV = \left| \frac{\overline{x}_1 - \overline{x}_2}{S_d} \right| \cdot \sqrt{\frac{N_1.N_2}{N_1 + N_2}}$$

Where $$S_d = \sqrt{\frac{(N_1 - 1).S^2_1 + (N_2 - 1)S^2_2}{N_1 + N_2 - 2}}$$

(For $N_1 = N_2 = N$, $f_1 = f_2$; $f = 2N - 2$ is valid)

Decision :

T (f, P = 95%) :

$TV \leq t$ (f, P = 95 %)	:	Random difference
$TV \leq t$ (f, P = 99 %)	:	Probable difference
$TV > t$ (f, P = 99 %)	:	Significant difference

4.5.27 Variance F-test

The F-test is used to test the inequality of two variances, determined from two independent data series.

$$TV = \frac{\text{Larger variance}}{\text{Smaller variance}}$$

$$TV = \frac{S_1^2}{S_2^2}$$

Decision :

$F\ (f_1, f_2, P = 95\%)$:

$TV \leq F\ (f_1, f_2, P = 95\ \%)$: Random difference

$TV \leq F\ (f_1, f_2, P = 99\ \%)$: Probable difference

$TV > F\ (f_1, f_2, P = 99\ \%)$: Significant difference

4.5.28 Grubbs Test for Outliers

To identify individual outliers the mean value and the standard deviation S are calculated from the analysis data. The analysis value x* having the greatest difference to the mean is tested according to the following conditional equation :

$$TV = \left| \frac{x^* - \bar{x}}{S} \right|$$

Decision :

$rM\ (N, P = 90\ \%)$:

$TV \leq rM\ (N, P = 90\%)$: random deviation

$TV \leq rM\ (N, P = 95\%)$: probable deviation

$TV > rM\ (N, P = 95\%)$: significant deviation

4.6 Sources of Error in Analytical Methods

Every analytical result contains unavoidable error. Knowledge of and attention to possible sources of error help to reduce considerably the occurrence of error and also locate more rapidly the causes of an error, which has appeared (trouble – shooting).

Error prevention is primarily achieved by optimizing the operational process. The better a laboratory is organized, the fewer errors can be expected. Optimal laboratory organization and quality assurance corroborate each other reciprocally.

If an analytical process is used routinely, then errors, which appear, may be categorized as follows :

1. Sample errors
2. Reagent errors

3. Reference material errors
4. Method errors
5. Calibration errors
6. Equipment errors
7. Signal registration and recording errors
8. Calculation errors
9. Transmission errors
10. Errors in the reporting of results.

One must also differentiate between three types of errors.

4.6.1 Classification of Errors

Gross Errors : A very large (gross) deviation appears in the results due to the presence of a gross error. Gross errors can appear randomly as so-called "outliers". Primary causes for these are random calculation errors, errors in transmission of information, misspellings, etc. Repeated incorrect preparation of standards and samples, incorrectly chosen analytical processes, systematic deviations from prescribed procedures (modification of analysis steps, use of incorrect equipment, systematic arithmetical errors, and so on, lead to gross errors for all results of one or more analysis series and can be detected by control analyses using an $\overline{x}$ -chart. It is difficult to distinguish between the gross errors mentioned above and systematic errors.

4.6.2 Systematic Errors

The analytical results show systematically high or low values. The accuracy of the results decreases.

4.6.3 Random Errors

The precision of the result decreases, the scatter increases.

A faulty result cannot always be categorized strictly as one type of error. A gross error is often only distinguishable from a systematic error by the extent of its influence on the result, or it consists of a combination of considerable systematic and random errors.

4.6.4 Systematic Trouble – Shooting

The identification and elimination of gross and systematic errors is primary routine of quality assurance. The process of identification of errors, include three steps :

- Awareness of changes in the analytical system and of unexpected incidents.

- Checking results for plausibility as a matter of course.
- Quality monitoring using control charts.

To a large extent successful trouble – shooting depends on experience and knowledge of the system. Therefore, sources of error and their elimination should be documented and discussed.

4.6.4.1 Analytical errors, which can be detected using statistical quality control methods

If an out of control situation appears on a control chart, then it must be conclude that the same error exists for the analysis of actual samples. A quick recognition and elimination of the existing error is absolutely necessary for the certainly of the analytical results.

Procedures for quick and successful trouble – shooting in analytical chemistry suggested in the following sections.

4.6.4.2 Elimination of Gross Errors

The control sample analysis is repeated while avoiding possible gross errors and strictly following established procedures. If the control sample results show that the process is again in control, then presumably the analysis protocol is not followed exactly for the previous analysis series or a gross error existed. The entire series of analyses must be repeated after elimination of this error.

On the other hand, if the analytical results of the control sample are error but reproducible, then a systematic error probably exists.

4.6.4.3 Elimination of Systematic Errors

To test for systematic errors, several different accuracy control samples are analysed if possible. In order to recognize reagent and method dependent errors, control samples should be used whose concentrations are distributed over the error measurement range. As a minimum an accuracy control sample should be used the lower and upper portions of the range. These additional control sample analyses will be worth the effort if the control charts used already indicate systematic error (trends). If a systematic error exists, i.e. if the results of the control sample predominantly above or below the expected values, then one should look for possible causes step by step using a source of error. Exchange experiments are recommended wherever possible; many errors can be detected quickly by exchanging individual reagents, equipment or personnel.

4.6.4.4 Improving Precision

Often, the dosage equipment and the work methods of the operators are causes of poor precision. In the worst case, the (Im) precision of the individual steps of a process and up according to the law or error propagation and are then known as the total (im) precision. If the total precision of a method is to be improved, then those analytical steps, which have the greatest influence on the total error of an analytical step, which have the greatest influence on the total error of an analytical process, must be identified.

Trouble – shooting schemes should if possible be created by the manufacturers of analytical instruments and analytical processes and be provided to users since it is impossible to create one generally applicable trouble – shooting scheme for all analytical processes.

Errors may also appear which cannot be detected using statistical quality assurance methods. These are mostly errors, which only affect one analysis and do not influence the next sample (e.g. gross., matrix or sample dependent errors, errors of transmission, and outcome or results). These errors can only be discovered using plausibility checks.

4.7 The four phase model of analytical quality assurance and application statistical methods for calibration of analytical methods :

4.7.1

A 4-phase model of analytical quality assurance using statistical methods for calibration of analytical methods is described below :

- ***Phase I :*** the quality characteristics of a new analytical process in need of calibration is determined and if necessary the process is improved and documented.
- ***Phase II :*** preparative quality control. An analytical process whose quality characteristics have already been documented is made operational for routine analysis. This includes achieving and maintaining sufficient analytical quality before routine analysis begins.
- ***Phase III :*** all internal laboratory quality assurance measures of routine analysis, accompanied by internal laboratory quality control and internal measures.
- ***Phase IV :*** external laboratory quality assurance in the form of inter-laboratory tests and external audits.

Only by tying together all analytical activities into a closed system of both internal and external laboratory quality assurance, reliability of analytical results can be guaranteed: these are on the one hand legally defensible and on the other hand, they can be used to make comparisons of trend experiments, establish registers of analytical values, etc.

4.7.2 Establishing a New Analytical Procedure

For allowing a new analytical procedure, especially one requiring calibration, for routine analysis, the individual steps need not only be determined but they must also be optimized if necessary, and the entire fundamental analytical procedure must be verified for its performance. The performance characteristics obtained in this way are documented and/or published with the description of the analysis and they form the basis for later quality assurance in routine analysis.

4.7.3 Statistical Methods for Establishing a New Analytical Procedure

Statistical methods are useful for fixing calibration, and precession measures in the establishment of new analytical process in Quality assurance.

4.8 Phase I of Analytical Quality Assurance-Testing of a New Analytical Method and Calibration

4.8.1

In the four phase model of Analytical quality assurance Phase I consists primarily the following five main steps ; (i) preparation of the calibration experiment, (ii) testing for linearity of the calibration function (iii) precision (variance homogeneity, absence of outliers, securing the lower bounds of the range), (iv) final determination of the calibration data and (v) testing for the influence of the individual process steps or for matrix effects on the calibration data (vi) Testing for the influence of time on the analytical process.

Phase I of analytical quality assurance lays the foundation for later routine analysis by providing quality data and includes (i) of the range tested, (ii) the coefficients of the calibration function, (iii) in the case of a first order calibration function ($y = a + bs$) axis intercept a and slope b (characteristic of the sensitivity of the analytical procedure (TV) in the case of a first order calibration function ($y = a + bx + cx^2$) axis intercept a coefficient b of the linear term, as well as the coefficient c of the quadratic term; the sensitivity E of the analytical process determined from the function. (v) The standard deviation of the procedure s_{xo} as an absolute measure of precision for the calibration and the process variation coefficient V_{xo} as a relative measure of precision.

In addition, the general evaluation of the analytical process also documents the limit of detection Lc Capability for detection XN Limit of quantitation XB Testing value x_a for the validation of a suitable range.

Proportional systematic errors related to certain matrices as well as an indication of the time dependency of the analytical results, the time required and other special remarks.

A flow chart giving the chronological order of various procedures to be followed in Phase I of four-phase analytical quality Assurance Model is shown in Fig. 4.1 (a) to (f).

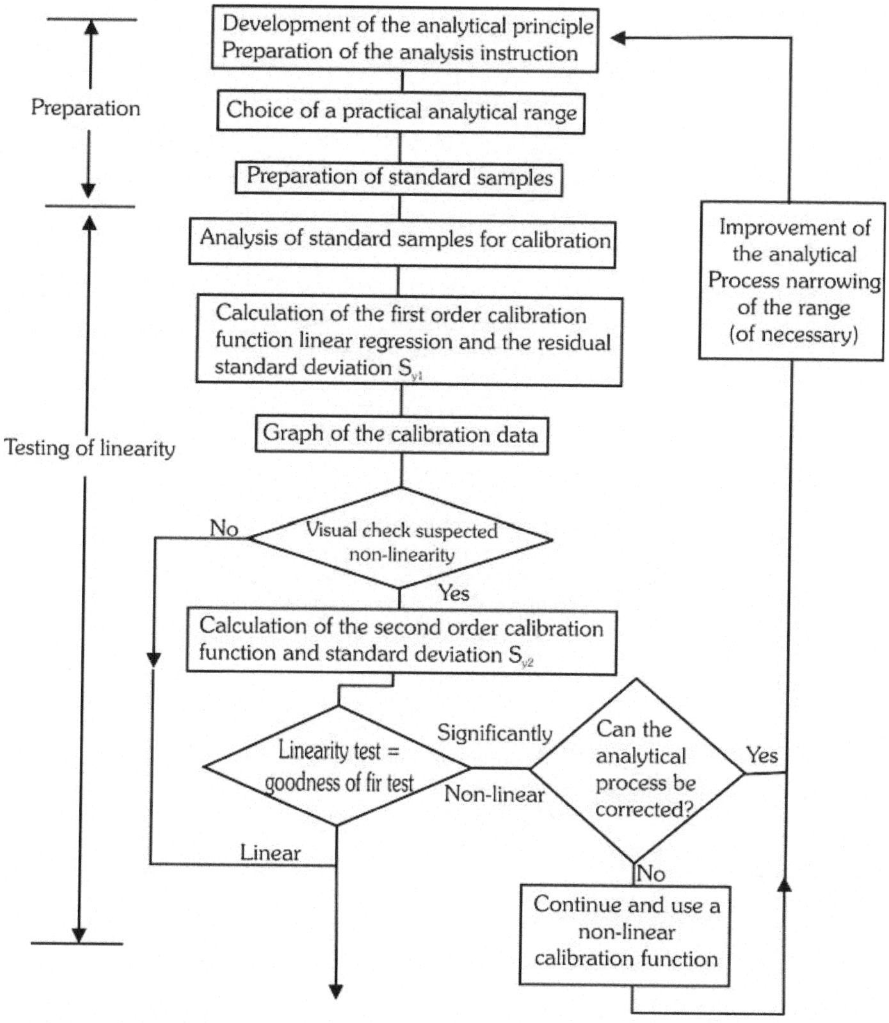

Figure 4.1 (a) Phase I of Analytical Quality Assurance model flow chart for documentation of the final calibration data.

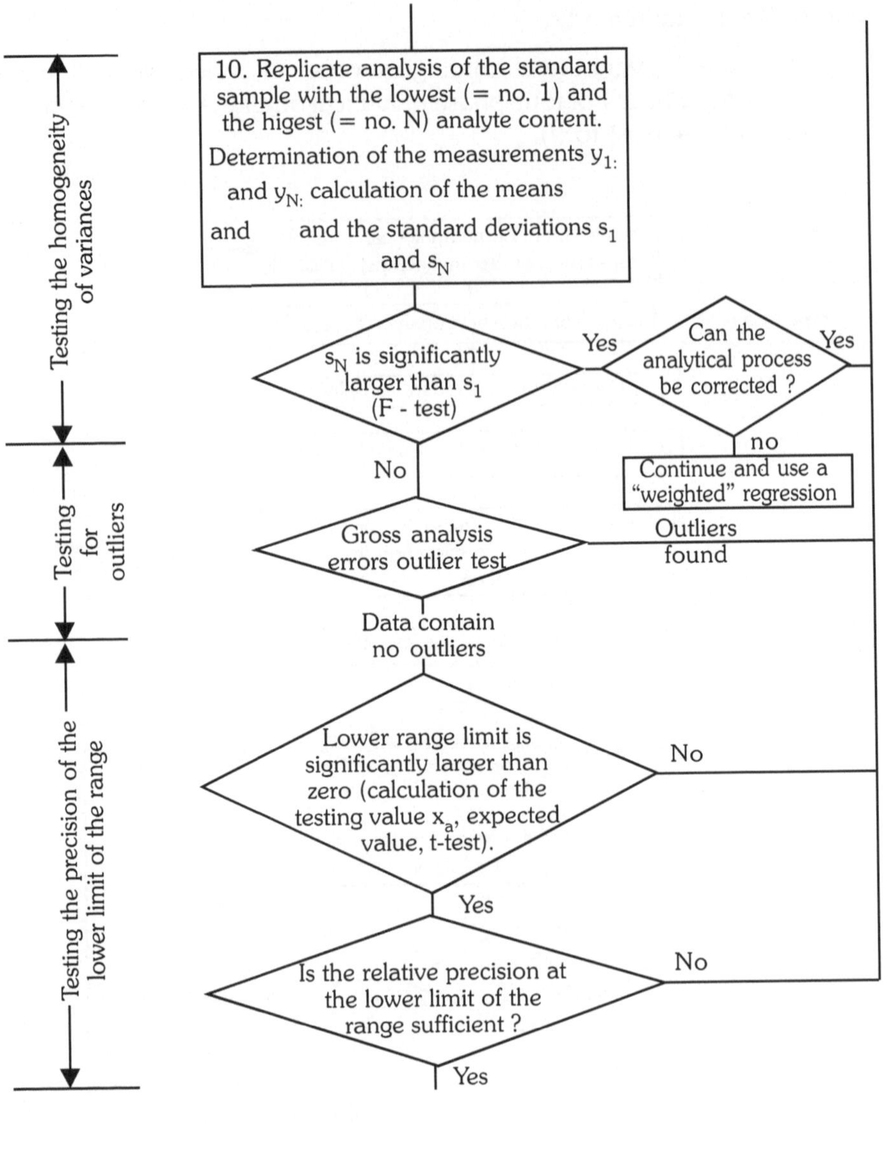

Figure 4.1 (b) Phase I of Analytical Quality assurance method Flow chart for testing for analytical method.

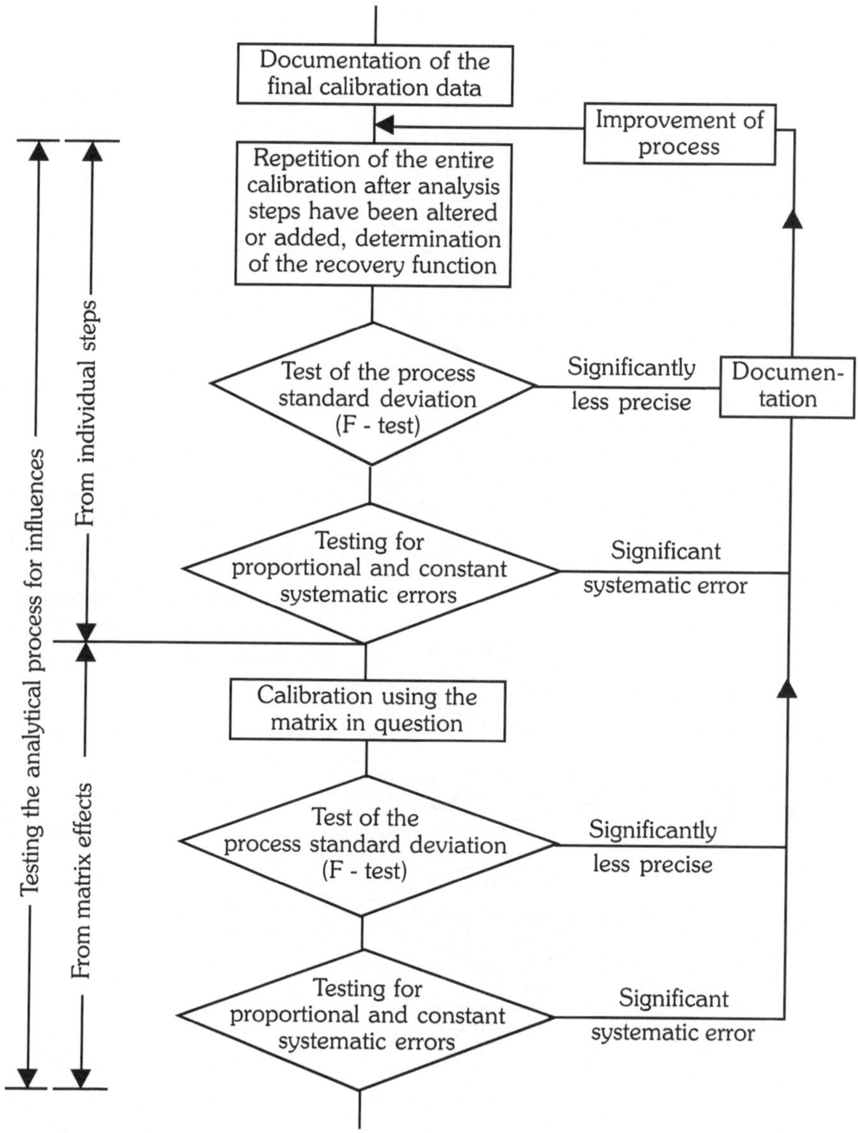

Figure 4.1 (c) Phase I of Analytical Quality Assurance model flow chart for establishing new analytical procedure.

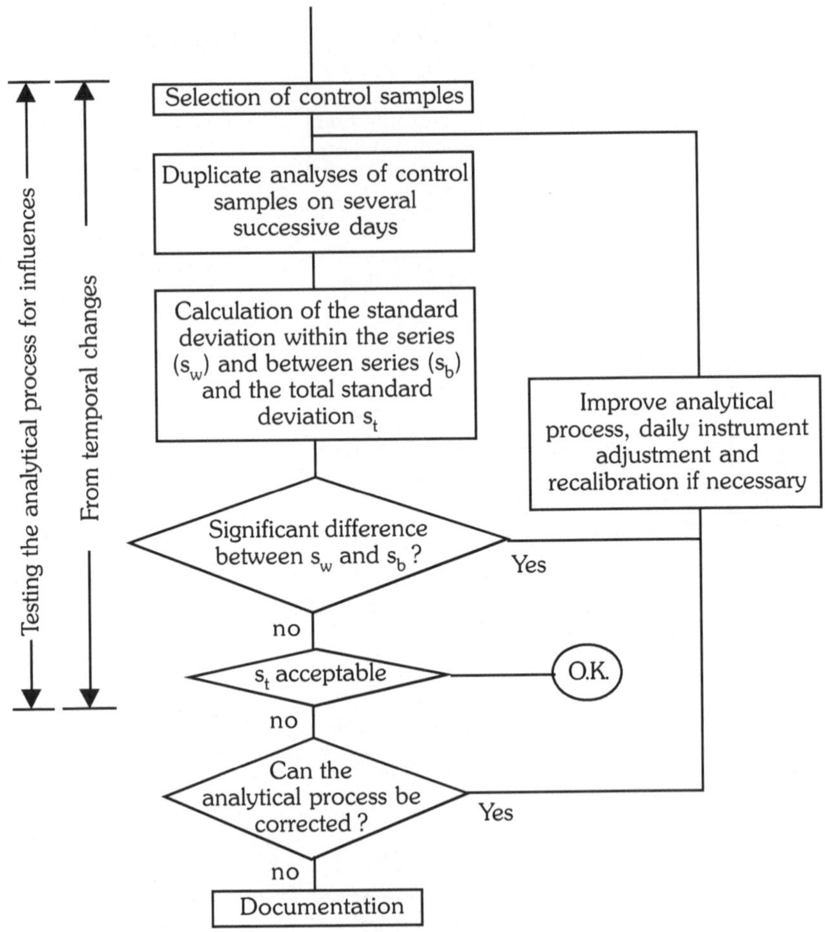

Figure 4.1 (d) Phase I of Analytical Quality assurance model flow chart for interference study.

4.8.2 Calibration of the Fundamental Analytical Procedure

For analytical processes which have to be calibrated, physical measurement data has to be converted into the analytical result using a calibration experiment.

The use of an analysis function

Analytical result = function of the observation or in mathematical notation :

$$\hat{x} = f\ (y)$$

(With y as the observation and $\hat{x}$ as the substance content/analytical result) is based on the application of the calibration function obtained from the calibration experiment observation = function of substance content or $\hat{y}$.

$$\hat{y} = f\ (x)$$

(with x = substance content of the standard sample and y = accompanying observation) and the precision data therefore for the determination of an unknown substance content in a sample. After solving for x the calibration function then becomes the analytical function, which, after inserting the observation of the tested sample y, gives the analytical result x.

A fundamental calibration represents the calibration of the fundamental analytical procedure, or in other words no sample preparation steps such as extraction or work up are performed, only standards in pure solvents (e.g. distilled water) are analyzed.

4.8.3 Establishment of an Analytical Range

Every calibration begins with the choice of a preliminary range as determined by :

(a) The objective of the application as related to practical conditions. This should cover a large range of applications. In addition, the mean of the range should be roughly equal to the sample concentration most often expected, as much as this is possible in individual cases.

(b) The technical possibilities.

(b1) The measured values at the lower end of the range must be significantly different from the process blank values. A lower range limit is only useful when it is at least the same or larger than the limit of detection of the procedure.

In addition, dilution concentration steps must be easily and flawlessly realized.

(b2) The required analytical precision must be achievable throughout the entire range. Since the imprecision of an analysis increases absolutely with increasing substance content, the range in question must not be chosen too large. If another range is necessary for routine analysis, then this should be divided into overlapping segments.

(b3) The analytical precision must be constant over the entire range (homogeneity of variances). Inhomogeneity of variances that is ignored can result in a large increase in the imprecision of analytical results obtained using the calibration function.

(b4) There must be a linear relationship between substance content and measured value.

In the case of inhomogeneity of variances or non-linearity, the chosen range must be reduced so as to fulfill these conditions, or more complicated calibration methods must be chosen, for example higher degree regression functions.

4.8.4 Preparation of Standard Samples

Requirements of a standard sample are : purity, either lack of a matrix or a defined matrix homogeneity.

- Representativeness : the substance to be analyzed must be present in the standard sample in ways comparable to those expected in later analysis samples, in other words compounds must be chemically similar, have the same oxidation state, etc.
  - Stability, ability to be preserved
  - Storage : samples may not be influenced by containers or outside conditions

Preparation of a standard sample :

- During preparation of a standard sample, the precision of the balance and volumetric equipment must be taken into account. Of the two, weighing is the most exact form of sample preparation and is therefore preferable to volumetric measurement.

A quality control check is necessary for this equipment.

- There should be no successive dilutions since this entails the risk of error propagation.

After establishing the preliminary range, N=6...10 standard samples are prepared so that their concentrations are distributed as equidistantly as possible over the entire chosen range.

4.8.5 Determination of the Calibration Function and Process Data

The preliminary first and second-degree calibration functions are calculated from the measured values obtained from these standard samples. The process data is necessary for further statistical tests.

Example : slope of the linear calibration function :

Substance content x : mg/l

Observation: peak height y : mm

Slope of the calibration function :

$$[\text{Peak height per substance content}] = \frac{\text{mm}}{\text{mg/l}}$$

Verification by calculation formulae :

$$\text{Slope} = \frac{\Sigma(x_i - \bar{x}).(y_i - \bar{y})}{\Sigma(x_i - \bar{x})^2}$$

$$= \frac{\Sigma\left\{\frac{\text{mg}}{1}.\text{mm}\right\}}{\Sigma\left\{\left(\frac{\text{mg}}{1}\right)^2\right\}}$$

$$= \frac{\Sigma\left\{\frac{\text{mg}}{1}\ .\ \text{mm}\right\}}{\Sigma\left\{\frac{\text{mg}}{1}\cdot\frac{\text{mg}}{1}\right\}}$$

$$= \left\{\frac{\text{mm}}{\text{mg/1}}\right\}$$

1. Generally the running index for summation signs (S) has been omitted. In these cases, the "I" forms the index and it runs from 1 to N.

Examples : $\Sigma\,(x_i - \bar{x})^2$ is equivalent to $\sum_{i=1}^{N}(x_i - \bar{x})^2$

4.8.6 Process Data for the Linear calibration Function

Regression analysis provides the calibration function with the characteristic data.

Slope (measure of sensitivity) : (Fig. 4.2).

$$b = \frac{\Sigma\left((x_i - \bar{x}) \cdot (y_i - \bar{y})\right)}{\Sigma(x_i - \bar{x})^2}$$

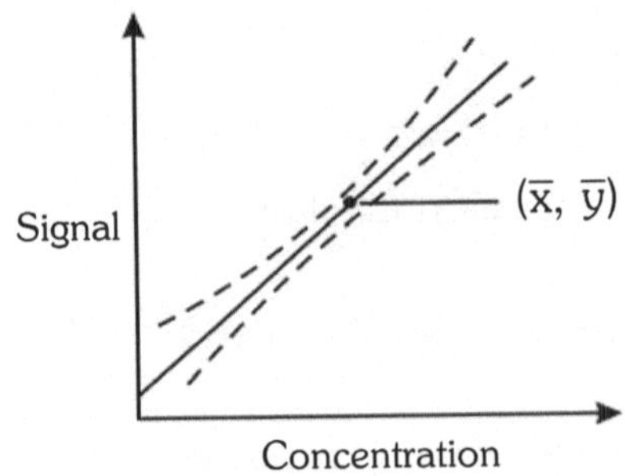

Figure 4.2 Linear calibration function (y = a +bx) with prognosis interval.

Sensitivity E :

The measure of sensitivity results from the change in the measured value caused by a change in the concentration values. If the calibration function for an analytical procedure is linear, then the sensitivity is constant over the entire range and is equivalent to the regression coefficient b. In the case of a curved calibration function, the sensitivity is still dependent on the given concentration value and is equivalent to the first derivative of the calibration function:

$$E(x) = b + 2c.x$$

As a process characteristic quantity it is recommended to express the sensitivity as the mean of the range x:

$$(\bar{x}) = b + 2c.\bar{x}$$

From this one can derive the process standard deviation:

Process standard deviation :

$$S_{xo} = \frac{S_y}{E(\bar{x})}$$

Relative process standard deviation :

$$V_{xo} = \frac{S_{xo}.100\%}{\bar{x}}$$

4.8.7 Verification of the Fundamental Calibrations

4.8.7.1 Verification of linearity

If possible, one should attempt to work with a first-degree calibration function. Second order calibration functions should only be used in justified exceptions.

4.8.7.2 Visual linearity test

The type of calibration function is most simply determined through graphic representation of the calibration data, including calibration line, and a subjective evaluation. If the measured data were highly precise and the result is obviously nonlinear, one may do without a special statistical test of linearity. In doubtful cases, however, the linearity should be verified mathematically.

The final documentation of a fundamental analytical process in phase I should include, in addition to the description of the analysis procedure, all relevant information above the analysis quality.

4.9 Phase II of Analytical Quality Assurance – Routine Preparation Quality Assurance

4.9.1 Preparation Quality Assurance

The objective of Phase II of 4-phase model of Analytical Quality Assurance is to make a verified analytical process available for routine analysis. Phase II is primarily of concern to the personnel who will be performing the routine analyses.

Phase II begins with a training phase of the analytical process and ends with the preparation of quality control charts for the routine use to follow. As the end of Phase II, the laboratory will not only have gained sufficient confidence and experience in the application of the analytical process in question, but it will also possess precision and reliability data which will serve during the routine period as a basis for quality assurance and control. This includes precision data such as the mean and the standard deviation of the analyses from control samples, the range of multiple analyses, the recovery rates of control samples, and especially the limits of reliability (scalier ranges, confidence intervals) within which limits future control analyses, or data derived there from, must lie.

The progressive steps to be followed for determining of an analytical procedure are presented in Fig. 4.3 (a) and 4.3 (b).

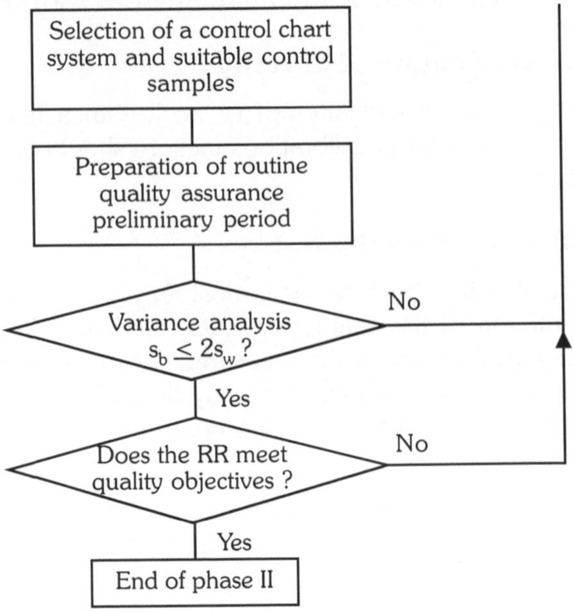

Figure 4.3 (a) Progression of phase II of analytical quality assurance model.

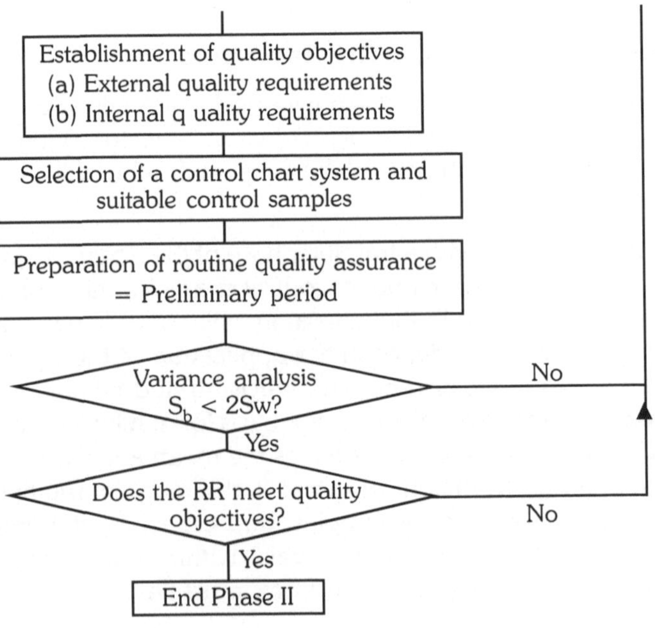

Figure 4.3 (b) Phase II of Analytical Quality Assurance model flow central for establishment of Quality Objectivities.

The procedure mainly depend on

(a) The substance to be determined
(b) Which chemical element or compound
(c) The physico-chemical state in which it occurs (dissolved, suspended, gaseous.
(d) Oxidation state, etc.
(e) The range of interest.
(f) The required accuracy (maximal acceptable systematic and random errors).
(g) The matrices to be investigated:
(h) The analytical equipment available, etc.

In addition, economical requirements (e.g. analysis time, capital and human resources, environmental and safety concerns, cost etc.) the analysis must be taken into account the Quality of data, which depends on the following characteristics of analytical procedures.

4.9.2 Specificity of the Procedure

Substances which cause errors (primarily systematic) in the determination of the analyte are known as interfering substances.

4.9.3 Selectivity of the Analytical Procedure

Many substances can exist in various physical and chemical forms (e.g. iron is found in soluble, colloidal or particle form, in different oxidation states and in complexes). It must be confirmed that the analytical procedure chosen covers all required forms, [16, 2].

4.9.4 Range

The range of the chosen analytical procedure must be fitted to the problem. Dilution or concentration steps which are not described in the protocol should only be admitted to the process after testing, if at all, since they can increase the inaccuracy of the entire process.

4.9.5 Calibration Function, Sensitivity and Precision of the Procedure

The calibration function determined by the process developer produces results related to the sensitivity, precision (residual standard deviation) and performance (process standard deviation) of the analytical procedure.

The user of the process performs the calibration as described in the protocol in his or her own laboratory and compares the data obtained, especially the process standard deviation, with the data provided.

4.9.6 Limit of Detection

The limit of detection of an analytical process is especially of interest if a substance is to be analyzed at the trace or ultra-trace level. In such situations the analyst must choose the process with the greatest sensitivity and lowest possible imprecision, that is the one with the lowest limit of detection.

The limit of detection of the fundamental analytical procedure should not be the sole consideration, since this ideal limit of detection is obtained by analyzing pure standard solutions, not including digestion, extraction, etc. The limit of detection for actual matrices can be considerably greater (by a factor of 5 to 10 times, based on experience). The reason for this is a possible negative influence of matrix components on the residual standard deviation s and the slope b of the calibration function. Therefore one must not only consider the results of the process developer with respect to matrix influences but also the actual limit of detection for one's own typical matrices using the method of standard addition.

4.9.7 Risk of Systematic Error

Since the process development cannot determine a recovery function for all possible types of matrices, the user should perform additional recovery experiments with his or her own matrices before beginning to use an analytical process in routine analysis.

4.9.8 Effort, Costs

Another criterion to be considered in the choice of an analytical process is the cost per analysis. The following factors are to be evaluated with respect to their effects on cost :

(a) *Time required :* This includes all the steps of sample preparation and analysis and can be determined from the analytical protocol. In addition to the time required for the analysis of actual samples, the following procedures also involve time, which must be included in the total determination:

(b) quality assurance measures:

(c) adjustment*

(d) calibration*

(e) training of personnel*

(f) control analysis within the framework of internal and external quality assurance*

(g) maintenance* including inspections and preventive maintenance of equipment and care of the laboratory and equipment

(h) quality assurance audits*

(i) evaluation and administrative work

All items marked with an asterisk* are nearly independent of the number of samples in an analysis series and can be termed "minimum effort"; this can influence the material requirements significantly. Rationalization and automatization are possible if the frequency of an analysis is high and can lower decisively the average time required per analysis.

- *Necessary equipment* : Acquisition of equipment for a new analytical process incurs investment and operating costs which are only economically justifiable at higher analysis frequency.
- *Material required* : in terms of quality, quantity and storage, the use of material can vary greatly between analytical processes.
- *Personnel required* : The number of persons and their qualifications must be considered and determined.
- *Type of application* : The effort involved in a process may vary depending on whether the process is used solely for qualitative analysis or if it can also be used for quantitative analysis, and if it is suitable for analyzing different types of matrices or if it possesses a very limited range of usage. The same is true for the evaluation of the range, which must not only be appropriate for practical use but should be as large as possible in order to minimize calibration and adjustment effort.
- In summary, the frequency of usage should be estimated for an analytical process. Processes, which are seldom used, can prove to be very cost intensive when the required quality assurance measures represent a large portion of the total costs.

4.9.9 The "Training" Phase of the Process

The so-called "training phase" includes the determination of the quality required as well as the testing and improvement of the quality achieved by the analytical process. Problems, which may appear in the analytical process itself, are to be investigated.

4.10 Phase III of Analytical Quality Assurance – Routine Quality Assurance

4.10.1 Routine Analysis in Analytical Quality Assurance

Includes both internal laboratory quality control and all external measures that are taken preventatively or as a result of alarming results. Routine refers here not only to the analyses, whose quality should continue to be guaranteed, but also to the quality assurance measures, which become a natural and routine portion of the analysis.

4.10.2 Quality Assurance Procedures

4.10.2.1 Internal quality assurance measures

Both of a statistical and process technological nature, are the responsibility of every laboratory which performs analyses whether on commission or within the framework of self-control. External quality assurance (Phase IV) can take place only in cooperation with the laboratories concerned. Preparation, organization and evaluation of interlaboratory (or round robin) tests are the business of external control laboratories, which should in addition assume the role of consultant.

Since the quality of analytical results is closely related to the quality of the instructions, then the latter should be clear, understandable and practically oriented, so that an analyst can follow unfamiliar instructions and obtain satisfactory results. The instructions are to be completed with the following information, for the most part obtained in Phase I :

(a) the substance to be analyzed (analyte)

(b) area of application, type of possible bulk (or gross) samples ~- tolerances (e.g. "add 6.0 ml ± 0.1 ml") in order to obtain the necessary precision at each analytical step

(c) measuring instructions, including physical quantity and unit of the measured value

(d) the procedure to determine the calibration function and the blank value

(e) the range

(f) calibration instructions: number, type, preparation of standard solutions

(g) coefficients of the calibration function with information about the linearity, sensitivity and residual standard deviation

(h) the process standard deviation

(i) the limit and capability of detection with information about how they were obtained including how many measurements were used.

(j) the relative imprecision at the lower limit of the range (CI_{rel} ($x_{:i}$) for later comparison with the required limit of quantitation

(k) instructions for the evaluation and description of the results

(l) frequently seen process errors and accompanying countermeasures

(m) quantitative information about interfering substances

(n) Qualitative and quantitative information about constant and proportional

(o) systematic deviations as well as their causes and elimination

(p) temporal stability (perishability) and storage information for samples, reagents, standard solutions and reference materials

(q) special notes;

- probable limits on the applicability of the process
- special procedures such as readjustment, recalibration, use of internal standards (including evaluation)
- determination and use of a blank
- notes about disposal of reagents and occupational safety
- literature references with further information (e.g. examples of applications)

The documentation is to be supplemented at a later time by means of interlaboratory test data, the routine analyses to follow and their respective quality assurance processes.

Quality assurance in Phase III includes all the components of analysis:

(a) the laboratory from the perspective of planning and equipping

(b) the equipment

(c) the personnel

(d) the analytical process

(e) spectrum of the process - requirements (including quality assurance requirements)

(f) the samples

(g) the reagents

(h) the "outcome", quality control and documentation

(i) the inclusion in an external quality assurance system

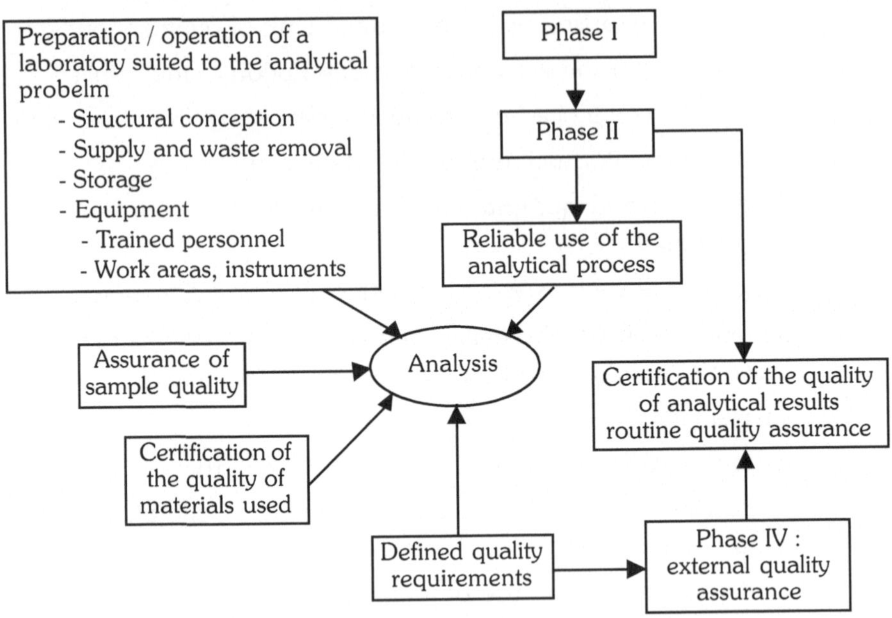

Figure 4.4 Phase III – Analytical quality assurance model. Routine quality assurance.

4.11 Phase IV : of Four Phase Analytical Quality Assurance Model - External Analytical Quality Assurance.

4.11.1

If the routine quality assurance measures are performed by analytical laboratories, then it is to be expected that these laboratories perform the analytical process in question reliably and results from these laboratories should be comparable for which external quality assurance resulting in general. The following are the different external measures used to check and prove a laboratory's quality system.

4.11.2 Analytical assessments in the form of interlaboratory trials with two objectives :

The assessment of the analytical procedure during the standardization process and the evaluation of the analytical performance of the laboratory in routine analysis and/or as part of an accreditation procedure.

Interlaboratory, or round-robin, tests can test the comparability of analytical results. The principle of interlaboratory tests is that identical samples are analyzed by different laboratories independently of one another, each under repeatable conditions. When these results are evaluated characteristic data are said to have been obtained under comparable or reproducible conditions.

Different types of samples may be used for interlaboratory test programs;

1. natural samples which have not been preserved
2. preserved natural samples
3. natural samples, originally having a low concentration of the analyte, which have been spiked
4. synthetic samples with problem-oriented matrix
5. synthetic samples without problem-oriented matrix

The "true value" (expected value) is only known for sample types 4 and 5. The mean analytical result, omitting outliers, is used primarily as the expected value (conventional accurate value) for the remaining sample types. Identical partial samples are taken from the inlet-laboratory test sample and are distributed to each of the participating laboratories.

There are two fundamentally different areas where interlaboratory testing is used: for process standardization for laboratory monitoring.

4.11.3 Interlaboratory Tests for Process Standardization

Interlaboratory tests performed inorder to formulate an official standard method document the current analytical status of the participating laboratories after a procedure has been established. They serve to determine the quality data of an analytical process: i.e. the characteristic process data such as recovery rate, comparative variation coefficient and repeat variation coefficient. In this way the reliability of an investigative method can be tested and documented.

Since participants in interlaboratory tests for the determination of characteristic process data are almost always renowned research, industrial and government laboratories, this may in some cases result in unrealistic data. For this reason, certain interest groups perform their own interlaboratory tests inorder to establish the characteristic process data of individual parameters for all laboratories involved in common measurement programs.

4.11.4 Interlaboratory Testing as Laboratory Monitoring

Interlaboratory tests are performed inorder to test, and ensure in the future, the performance of participating laboratories and the comparability of their analytical results. Without comparable analytical results (from all participating laboratories assured over the entire time span) no meaningful description of an entity, a body of water for instance, can be made.

The comparison of analytical results is even more important if the quality of results is doubted in a disagreement (e.g. for the calculation of sewage fees).

In this case, the respective laboratory must be able to document that the required precision and accuracy was maintained on the day that the result was produced. That means that the laboratory must be included in an internal and external quality assurance system. The AQA of a laboratory is comprised of participation in interlaboratory tests.

4.11.5 Audits

Audits may be performed internally or externally. Internal audits are part of the Analytical quality assurance system. They are carried out regularly by a competent independent member of the staff (in areas where he or she is not personally involved) or by an external consultant. The aim of an internal audit is the assessment of the current Analytical quality assurance system and the proposal of necessary corrective measures and alterations. Besides scheduled internal audits additional partial or total quality audits should be performed in cases of severe quality problems or preceding an important external audit.

4.11.6 External Audits Serve Different Purposes

- Certification audits are performed by an official laboratory accreditation body [EN 45003] to prove the conformity of a product, a service or a procedure with given standards. For example, a quality assurance system may be certified according to one of the ISO or EN standards. In the field of chemical analyses and measurements however, accreditation has become more important than certification.

- Accreditation audits according to EN 45002 are performed in order to obtain accreditation for all work performed by the laboratory or only for selected analytical procedures.
- The permission to work in a special, legally defined field (so called regulated field) or
- The proof of qualified analytical work as a recommendation for clients (deliberate accreditation).

  Accreditation according to EN 45002 is valid in every EU member country.
- Assessment of performance by a client's auditor as part of a larger contract.
- Official audit of chemical or pharmaceutical manufacturer laboratories by a local or national authority in order to obtain permission for production or sales. This kind of audit takes place according to the OECD code on Good Laboratory Practice or to the WHO Good Manufacturing Practice (GMP) Guide for pharmaceutical products or to national regulations (e.g. FDA and EPA in the USA).

The procedure for an internal or external quality audit in an analytical laboratory can be based on different strategies:

The process-oriented audit follows the chronology of work on a sample either forward, from sampling to report of results, or backward. The complaint-oriented audit reviews the most recent complaints and examines the handling of complaints and how information from complaints is used for quality improvement. The documentation-oriented audits checks all documentation and procedures according to the quality manual.

The system-oriented audit checks the quality management system according to organograms, relationships, responsibilities, and flow charts for material and information.

Execution and evaluation of interlaboratory (or round robin) tests.

Interlaboratory tests are executed and evaluated according to the following standard methods :

- ISO 5725 (Fig. 4.5).

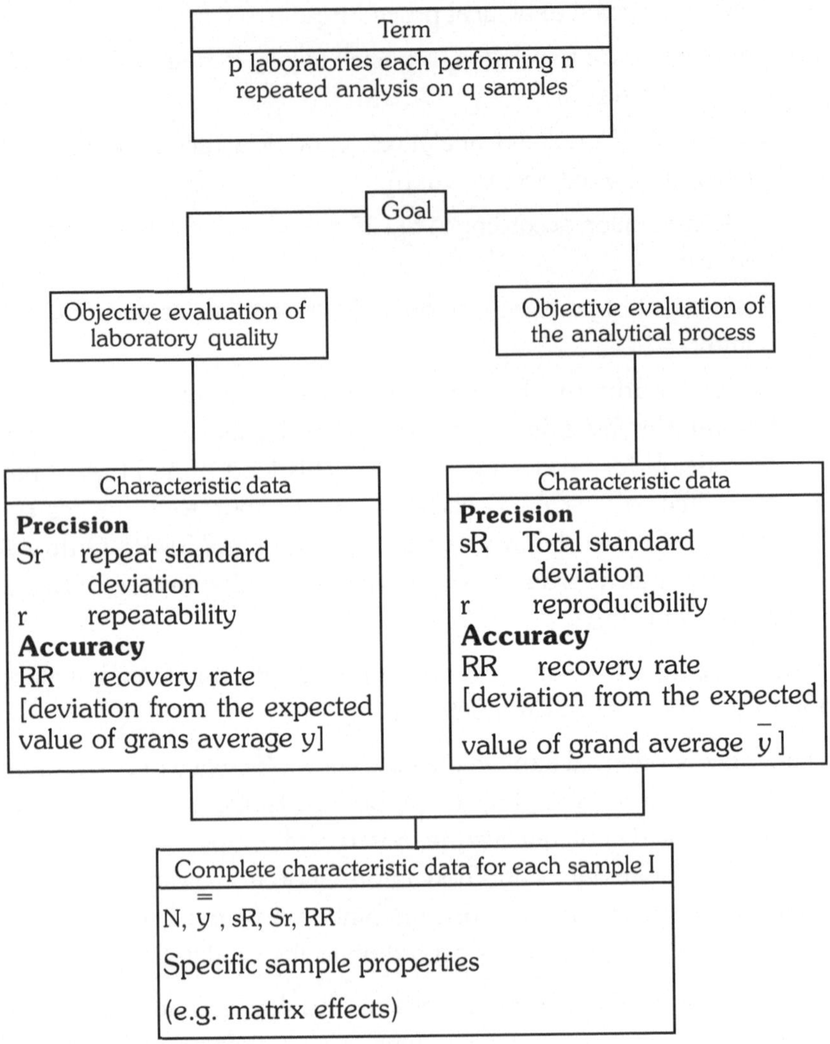

Figure 4.5 Interlaboratory test evaluation according to ISO 5725–2; characteristic data.

Summary

The objective of analytical work is the achievement of reliable analytical results of a defined quality. Quality characteristics of analytical processes are therefore :

Specificity : the ability of an analytical process to register only the desired analyte, while other components or characteristics present in the sample (known as the matrix) do not influence the result.

Sensitivity : the change in measured value per change in analyte concentration.

Accuracy : in the sense of both trueness (lack of systematic errors) and precision (measurement of differences between results, as obtained by repeated use of an established analytical process on the same sample, precision is caused by random errors).

Quality of analytical processes and results

The appropriate analytical process for obtaining the answer to a specific question need not always be the scientifically "best" procedure. However, it is important that the results of an analysis, obtained through adherence to legal regulations, should if necessary be defensible in court, or in other words legally binding.

Statistical methods for analytical procedure

Statistical methods are used for planning, interpretation and assessment of the data generated by analytical method.

Reliability

Quality under set application conditions during or after a set time period.

Measurement principles

Characteristic physical! Properties, which are used for measurement (e.g. photometry).

Measurement methods

Practical application of measurement principles

Direct : obtaining measured values by immediate comparison with a reference quantity (e.g. volume measurements)

Indirect : reduction of measured values to different physical quantities (i.e. operational parameters)

Analytical principle

Refers only to the measurement and the evaluation of measured values

Analytical procedure

Refers only to the determination of a defined substance and the evaluation of measured values.

Analytical method

An analytical process is a combination of processes like preparation (object dependent) which is shown schematically in techniques (sample taking, sample preparation). Principle, analytical procedure and analytical method :

Standard methods

A standard method is an acknowledged analytical method according to an international or national standard or guideline or to a given legal statute, synonyms for standard methods; Arbitration methods

Reference methods

Standard methods : which may be national standard procedures, or international (e.g. ASTM, ISO, ECCLES, CEN, IUPAC, etc) guidelines and standards, or procedures described by legal regulations. Standard methods represent the accepted latest state of engineering; their use may be prescribed and/or obligatory within a framework of regulations and guidelines.

Comparable laboratory procedures : quantitative analytical processes which vary in procedure from standard methods, but whose equivalence is verified using standard methods.

Other quantitative analytical procedures which have various uses and objectives in the laboratory outside of governmentally regulated areas. These also include the latest analytical procedures for which standards have not yet been established.

Field methods : analytical process which can be performed outside the laboratory. With the aid of objective measurement methods, field methods can bring quantitative or semi-quantitative results depending on previous handling of the sample and quality assurance procedures.

Orientation tests assess subjectively; they can qualitatively prove the presence of a certain substance and allow a concentration estimate to be made which is accurate to within one order of magnitude.

True value

Real (theoretical) characteristic value under conditions prevailing during the analysis.

Note : The true value is often an ideal value because it can only be determined if all errors in the results could be avoided, or a is a result of theoretical considerations.

Conventional true value

A value for the sake of comparison, whose deviation from the true value is considered to be negligible for comparative purposes. The conventional true value is an approximation for the true value. If can be obtained from international, national or usage norms, from reference materials or standard methods *(e. g.* on *the* basis of specially organized experi*ments*). There are several *terms, which* are used as synonyms of "conventional true value". Examples are "expected value" and "target value". These terms are ambiguous and should be avoided.

Expected value

The mean experimental result obtained using a continuously repeated experimental process under established conditions.

Actual value

An analytical result obtained momentarily, generally differentiated from the "expected value" (conventional true value) by the presence of systematic and/or coincidental error.

Accuracy

Accuracy is a qualitative term for the extent of the approximation of analytical results to the reference value, which may be cither the true, real or expected value depending on definition or agreement.

Accuracy is therefore a generic term for precision and trueness.

- The determining factor for the overall error is the largest individual error.
- The random error may be decreased by a factor 0^ by repeating the analyses N times.
- Systematic error may only be eliminated by the elimination of its cause.

Precision

Precision is a qualitative term for the extent of the mutual approximation of analytical results independent from one another by repeated use of a set analytical process under defined conditions.

The conditions under which analytical results are obtained must be reported exactly. One should notice the distinction between repeatability and reproducibility.

Repeatability, within run (or batch) precision

Repeatability is a qualitative term for the extent of reciprocal approximation of analytical results under repeat conditions. The terms "precision under repeat conditions" and/or "serial repeated Precision" may also be used.

Repeat conditions : Conditions for obtaining independent analytical results consisting of the repealed use of a set analytical process or method on the same object (same material, same sample) by the same observer in small time intervals (immediately following each other) with the same equipment (as well as identical supplies and other materials) in the same place (same laboratory).

Reproducibility

Reproducibility is a qualitative term for the extent of reciprocal approximation of analytical results under comparable conditions. The terms "precision under comparable conditions" and/or "precision from lab to lab" are sometimes used in everyday speech.

Analytical specificity

Analytical specificity is the ability of an experimental process to register only analyte, whereby other components or characteristics present in the sample do not influence the analytical result

Analytical sensitivity

Sensitivity describes the ability of an experimental method to differentiate between related values (e.g. concentrations). It indicates to which degree a value changes depending upon the signal of the measuring system and can be quantified using the slope of the calibration curve.

Validation

Validation is the total testing procedure if an analytical method is free of-random and systematic errors, not only within calibration but also and especially free of interferences when analyzing real samples. National regulations may establish official validation for special measurement instruments, consisting of testing done by the appropriate authorities carried out according to sit regulations. A validation seal may also be affixed.

Calibration

The calibration of a system is the determination and establishment of a functional relationship between a numerical or measurable quantity and a concentration to be determined (activity, frequency, etc.) from data, which are generally subject to random errors.

Adjustment

Adjustment is setting or aligning a measuring instrument so that measurement errors are kept as snail as possible or that the total measurement error does not exceed the limits of error.

Level of significance P

The level of significance P denotes the relative safety of a "statistical decision".

Bulk sample

A bulk sample is one taken on the spot, whose content r of a substance is to be determined quantitatively, the analytical result x therefore represents an approximation of the true value r.

Analytical sample

An analytical sample is a sample which is obtained from the bulk sample after a work-up (e.g. disintegration, extraction, etc.) and, if necessary, dilution (or concentration) and which will be used for the actual measuring process. An analytical sample is therefore identical with a bulk sample if the original sample may be used directly in the measuring process without work-up and dilution (or concentration).

Measurement sample

A measurement sample is a sample whose content of analyte may be measured directly. A measurement sample is normally obtained from an analytical sample by the addition of a series of reagents. Measurement samples and analytical samples are therefore identical when no reagents are added to the analytical sample.

Mean t-test

A test of the statistical difference between two means (X_1, X_2) obtained from two independent series of analyses (normal distribution assumed or required). A testing value TV is calculated and compared with the threshold value t from the t-Table:

Variance F-test

The F-test is used to test the inequality of two variances, determined from two independent data series

Grubbs test for outliers

To identify individual outliers the mean value x and the standard deviation s are calculated from the analysis data. The analysis value x* having the greatest difference to the mean is tested according to the following conditional equation:

Sources of error in analytical methods

Every analytical result contains unavoidable error. Knowledge of and attention to possible sources of error help to reduce considerably the occurrence of error and also locate more rapidly the causes of an error, which has appeared (trouble – shooting).

Error prevention is primarily achieved by optimizing the operational process. The better a laboratory is organized, the fewer errors can be expected. Optimal laboratory organization and quality assurance corroborate each other reciprocally.

If an analytical process is used routinely, then errors, which appear, may be categorized as follows:

- Sample errors, Reagent errors, Reference material errors, Method errors, Calibration errors, Equipment errors, Signal registration and recording errors, Calculation errors, Transmission errors, Errors in the reporting of results
- One must also differentiate between three types of errors.
- A 4-phase model of analytical quality assurance using statistical methods for calibration of analytical methods involves the following points :
- **Phase I :** the quality characteristics of a new analytical process in need of calibration is determined and if necessary the process is improved and documented.
- **Phase II :** preparative quality control. An analytical process whose quality characteristics have already been documented is made operational for routine analysis. This includes achieving and maintaining sufficient analytical quality before routine analysis begins.
- **Phase III :** all internal laboratory quality assurance measures of routine analysis, accompanied by internal laboratory quality control and internal measures.
- **Phase IV :** external laboratory quality assurance in the form of inter-laboratory tests and external audits.

Only by tying together all analytical activities into a closed system of both internal and external laboratory quality assurance, reliability of analytical results be guaranteed the phase of analytical quality assurance and application statistical methods for calibration of analytical method, these are on the one hand legally defensible and on the other hand, they can be used to make comparisons of trend experiments, establish registers of analytical values, etc.,

Questions

1. Define quality characteristics of analytical process like specificity, sensitivity and accuracy?
2. Name the tasks required in general in any analytical procedures?
3. Based on the observation, effort and degree of the information required how to categorize analytical process?
4. Discuss the precautions required during an analytical process?
5. Discuss queries and process like analytical procedures, analytical principle and analytical information in an analytical method systematically?
6. Explain the various statistical methods used for establishing new analytical procedure.
7. Explain various types of error in analytical methods and discuss thoroughly?
8. What are the various methods, which can be used for elimination of errors?
9. Explain the various components of 4 phase model of analytical quality assuarance?

5

Interpretation of Good Manufacturing Practice-Guide for Active Pharmaceutical Ingredients

5.1 Quality Management in Pharmaceutical Industry

The basic elements of Quality Management in a pharmaceutical industries are:

(a) Appropriate infrastructure and quality system, encompassing the organizational structure, procedures, processes, and resources;

(b) Systematic actions necessary to ensure adequate confidence that a product (or service) will satisfy given requirements for quality. The totality of these actions are termed as "quality assurance".

The concepts of Quality Assurance, Good Manufacture Practice (GMP), and Quality Control are interrelated aspects of quality management, which are described here inorder to emphasize their relationship and their fundamental importance to the production and control of pharmaceutical products.

5.1.1 Quality Assurance in Pharmaceutical Industry

Quality assurance is the activity for providing, to all concerned, the evidence required to establish confidence to customer that the quality function is being performed adequately. Under WHO GMP text, Quality Assurance has been defined as under:

"Quality Assurance is a wide range concept covering all matters that individually or collectively influence the quality of a product. It is the totality of the arrangements made with the object of ensuring that pharmaceutical products are of required quality meeting their intended use",

With reference to pharmaceutical industry Quality Assurance will be done in which implementation of Good Clinical Practices (GCP), Good Manufacturing Practices (GMP), Good Laboratory Practices (GLP), exist. Thus Quality Assurance can be represented as,

Quality assurance =GCP + GMP + GLP

WHO GMP text also states that the system of Quality Assurance appropriate to the manufacture of Pharmaceutical products should ensure that:

- Pharmaceutical products are designed and developed in a way that takes account of the requirements of GMP and other associated codes such as those of Good laboratory practice (GLP) and Good clinical practice (GCP).
- Production and control operations specified in a document form should be adopted for implementation.

  This is a code governing the testing of chemicals to obtain data on their properties and ensuring safety with respect to human health and environment. It is different from that described in Good Laboratory Practices Thirtieth Report of the WHO Expert committee on specifications for Pharmaceutical Preparation. (WHO Technical Report Series No.748. 1998)
- Managerial responsibilities are clearly specified in job descriptions.
- Arrangements are made for the manufacture, supply, and use of the correct starting and packaging materials.
- All necessary controls on starting materials, intermediate products, and bulk products and other in-process controls, calibrations, and validations are carried out.
- The finished product is correctly processed and checked according to the defined procedures.
- Pharmaceutical products are not sold or supplied before the authorized persons have certified that each production batch has been produced and controlled in accordance with the requirements of the marketing authorization and any other regulations relevant to the production, control and release of pharmaceutical products.

- Satisfactory arrangements exist to ensure, as far as possible, that the pharmaceutical products are stored by the manufacturer, distributed and subsequently handled so that quality is maintained throughout their shelf-life.
- There should be a procedure for self-inspection and /or quality audit that regularly appraises the implementation effectiveness and applicability of the quality assurance system for intended use.

The manufacturer must assume responsibility for the quality of the pharmaceutical products to ensure that they are fit for their intended use, comply with the requirements of the marketing authorization and do not place patients at risk due to inadequate safety, quality, or efficacy. The attainment of this quality objective is the responsibility of Top Management and requires the participation and commitment of staff in many different departments and at all levels within the company, the company's suppliers, and the distributors. To achieve the quality objective reliably there must be a comprehensively designed and correctly implemented system of quality assurance incorporating GMP and Quality Control. It should be a fully documented system and its effectiveness monitored periodically. All parts of the quality assurance system should be adequately staffed with competent personnel, and should have suitable and sufficient premises, equipment, and facilities.

5.2 Good Manufacturing Practices for Pharmaceutical Products (GMP)

5.2.1 Good Manufacturing Practice is that part of quality assurance which ensures that products are consistently produced and controlled to the quality standards appropriate to their intended use and as required by the marketing authorization. GMP rules are directed primarily to diminishing the risks, inherent in any pharmaceutical production, that cannot be prevented completely through the testing of final products, such risks are essentially of two types: cross contamination (in particular by unexpected contaminants) and mix-ups (confusion) caused by false labels being put on containers. Under GMP :

(a) All manufacturing processes are clearly defined, systematically reviewed in the light of experience, and shown to be capable of consistently manufacturing pharmaceutical products of the required quality that comply with their specifications;

(b) Critical steps of manufacturing processes and any significant changes made to the processes are validated;

(c) All necessary facilities are provided, including:
   (i) Appropriately qualified and trained personnel;
   (ii) Adequate premises and space;
   (iii) Suitable equipment and services;
   (iv) Correct materials, containers, and labels;
   (v) Approved procedures and instructions;
   (vi) Suitable storage and transport; and
   (vii) Adequate personnel, facilities, and equipment for in-process controls under the responsibility of the production management;

(d) Instructions and procedures, are written in clear and unambiguous language, specifically applicable to the facilities provided;

(e) Operators are trained to carry out procedures correctly:

(f) Records are made (manually and/or by recording instruments) during manufacture to show that all the steps required by the defined procedures and instructions have in fact been taken and that the quantity and quality of the product are as expected; any significant deviations are fully recorded and investigated;

(g) Records covering manufacture and distribution, which enable the complete history of a batch to be traced, are retained in a comprehensible and accessible form;

(h) The proper storage and distribution of the products minimizes any risk to their quality;

(i) A system is available to recall any batch of product from sale or supply;

(j) Complaints about marketed products are examined; the causes of quality defects investigated, and appropriate measures taken in respect of the defective products and to prevent recurrence.

A. Manufacturing : Include all operations of

(i) Receipt of materials.
(ii) Transportation of materials.
(iii) Production operation.
(iv) Packaging operation.
(v) Repackaging operation.
(vi) Labeling operation.
(vii) Re-labeling operation.
(viii) Quality control function.

(ix) Release activity.

(x) Storage activity.

(xi) Distribution of APIs and the related controls.

B. "Current good manufacturing practices" and "good manufacturing practices" are equivalent. Good manufacturing practice is the bare regulatory document. Current word refers applicability of amendments and changes as and when applicable.

C. Applicability :

Applies to manufacturing of Active Pharmaceutical Ingredients (APIs) for use in human drug (medicinal) products including sterile APIs.

D. Covers APIs that are manufactured by

(i) Chemical synthesis.

(ii) Extraction Process.

(iii) Cell culture/Fermentation Process.

(iv) Recovery from natural sources.

(v) Any combination of these processes.

E. Exclusions : This document does not address

(i) All vaccines Operations.

(ii) Whole cells process.

(iii) Whole blood and plasma Process.

(iv) APIs derived from plasma Process.

(v) Medical gases.

(vi) Radio pharmaceuticals.

5.2.2 Quality Management

A. Principles :

(i) Recording of all quality related activities.

(ii) Deviations (Critical deviations must be investigated, and conclusions must be documented)

(iii) Procedure for quality related complaints.

(iv) Procedure for product recall.

(v) Procedure for regulatory communications.

(vi) QC/QA should be independent of production unit.

(vii) Materials release responsibility must be specified and responsibility must be with quality unit.

B. Responsibilities of quality unit :

(i) Involvement in all quality related matters.

(ii) Review and approval of quality related documents.

(iii) Release or reject of all materials.

(iv) Review of Batch Manufacturing Records (BMRs) before release of APIs for distributions.

(v) Investigation of critical deviations.

(vi) Approval of specifications.

(vii) Approval of master production instructions.

(viii) Approval of procedures.

(ix) Conducting internals audits (self-inspections).

(x) Approval of contract manufacturing activities.

(xi) Approval of changes.

(xii) Review and approval of validation protocols and reports.

(xiii) Investigation and resolving of quality related complaints.

(xiv) Maintenance and calibration of critical equipments.

(xv) Material testing results documentation

(xvi) Stability studies monitoring

(xvii) Product quality reviews

(xviii) Master validation plan

(xix) Approval of vendors.

C. Responsibilities of production unit :

(i) Preparation and review of BMRS

(ii) Carrying out production as per BMRS instructions

(iii) Review of completed BRMS

(iv) Reporting of deviations, investigation of critical deviations and recording of conclusions.

(v) Maintenance of production equipments.

(vi) Calibration of production equipments.

(vii) Make sure production premises and equipments are well maintained.

(viii) Preparation and review of validation plans, protocols and reports.

(ix) Evaluation of product, process, equipment changes.

(x) Equipment qualification.

D. Internal Audit :

Self-inspection programme. This function should be organised by quality unit at pre-defined intervals. Audits must be performed by independent personnel not connected with the activity being audited. Connective actions must be renewed and approved by quality unit.

E. Product Quality Review :

(i) Review of critical inprocess and critical API test results.
(ii) Review of failed batches.
(iii) Review of critical deviations and investigation reports.
(iv) Review of changes made in the process, method, equipments or site.
(v) Review of results of stability data.
(vi) Review of quality related returns, complaints and recalls.
(vii) Review of adequacy of corrective actions.
(viii) Review of product review evaluation.
(ix) Review of product/Process development.
(x) Review of customer's requirements and expectations.
(xi) Review of current regulatory status.
(xii) Conducted at least annually.

5.2.3 Personnel

A. Personnel Qualifications :

(i) Appropriate and adequate number of people to perform the operations.
(ii) Responsibilities must be documented.
(iii) CGMP training, records, periodical evaluation and effectiveness of training must be documented.
(iv) Re-training can be planned as applicable.

B. Personnel Hygiene :

(i) Personnel should practice good sanitation and health habits.
(ii) Should wear clean clothing, head, face, hand and arm should be covered when required.
(iii) Avoid direct contact with intermediates or APIs.
(iv) Smoking, eating, drinking, chewing and storage of food should be restricted to areas different from manufacturing site.
(v) Personnel suffering from diseases, illness or having open lesions should be avoided in activities.

C. Consultants :

(i) Should possess sufficient education, training and experience in the field of activity.

(ii) Records should be maintained (name, address, qualifications and type of services offered).

5.2.4 Building and Facilities

A. Design and construction :

(i) Building and facilities must be suitable for the operation and should include adequate space.

(ii) Flow of material and personnel (to prevent mix-ups and contamination) should be independent

(iii) Defined areas for receipt, identification, sampling, pending release or rejection, holding of rejected materials, storage for release materials, production, packing, labeling operations control and laboratory operations.

(iv) Washing facilities for personnel (hot and cold water) must be provided.

(v) Separate washing and toilet facilities, easily accessible to manufacturing operations and separate change rooms for personnel should be in place.

(vi) Separate laboratory facilities and must be delinked from production areas.

B. Utilities :

(i) Utilities that could impact on production quality (e.g. steam, gases, and compressed air) should be qualified.

(ii) Adequate ventilation and exhaust system should be in place.

(iii) If air is recirculated to production areas, appropriate measures should be taken to control risk of contamination and cross-contamination.

(iv) Pipelines must be maintained and suitably identified.

(v) Drains should be of adequate size and should be provided with an air break or a suitable device to prevent back-siphonage.

C. Water :

(i) Process water should meet national or WHO standards.

(ii) If potable water is insufficient to assure API quality, tighter chemical, microbiological and endotoxins water quality specifications are necessary.

(iii) Where water treatment is installed, the water system must be validated and maintained with appropriate action limits.

(iv) Where non-sterile API is intended for further processing to produce a sterile drug product, then water used in the final isolation and purification steps should be monitored and controlled for.

(a) TMC (Total Microbial Content) to be estimated to assess safety

(b) Objectionable organisms and endotoxins should be absent.

D. Containment :

(i) Dedicated production areas for penicillin's or cephalosporins.

(ii) Dedicated areas should be considered for high toxic materials, steroids, and cytotoxic agents.

(iii) Should avoid personnel, materials movement from one dedicated areas to the other.

(iv) Highly toxic non-pharmaceutical materials (pesticides or herbicides) should be separate from the APIs.

E. Lighting :

(i) Lighting should be adequate to facilitate cleaning, maintenance and to perform operations.

F. Sewage and Refuse :

(i) Separate storage and disposal areas for the waste must be provided.

G. Sanitation and Maintenance :

(i) Building should be in clean condition.

(ii) Cleaning procedures for facilities and equipment must be established.

(iii) Use of rodenticiedes, insecticides, fungicides, fumigation agents and cleaning agents must be justified

5.2.5 Process Equipment

A. Design and Constructions :

(i) All equipment should be of

(a) Appropriate design

(b) Adequate size and

(c) Suitability located for cleaning, sanitation and maintenance.

(ii) Equipment material of construction should not alter the quality of processed materials.

(iii) Production materials should be qualified.

(iv) All the equipment should be qualified.

(v) Lubricants, heating fluids or coolants should not come into contact with materials, wherever possible food grade lubricants and oils should be used.

(vi) Closed equipment should be used to avoid or minimize contamination.

(vii) For equipment and critical installation, current drawing should be maintained.

B. Equipment maintenance and cleaning :

(i) Preventive maintenance of equipment (SOP, records) should be established.

(ii) Written equipment cleaning procedures should be in place. The procedure should include the minimum requirements and should be not be limited to:

(a) The responsibilities for cleaning of equipment

(b) Cleaning schedules, sanitizing schedules.

(c) Complete description of cleaning agents.

(d) The areas identified for cleaning.

(e) Removal of previous batch materials and their limits.

(f) Instructions to protect the cleaning equipment from contamination prior to use.

(g) Inspection of equipment for cleanliness before use.

(h) Establish the maximum time that may elapse between the completion of process and equipment cleaning.

(iii) All the equipment should be cleaned, stored and sanitized to prevent contamination.

(iv) Campaign production equipment should be cleaned to prevent contaminants and objectionable microorganism.

(v) Non-dedicated equipment should be cleaned between productions of different materials to prevent contamination.

(vi) Acceptance criteria for residues and cleaning agents should be defined and justified.

(vii) Equipment cleaning status should be identified.

C. Calibration :

(i) Control, weighing, measuring and monitoring and test equipment should be calibrated as per the calibration procedures and schedules.

(ii) Equipment calibration should be carried out using primary standards.

(iii) Calibration status records should be maintained.

(iv) Calibration status of equipment should be maintained.

(v) Equipment that do not meet calibration criteria should not be used.

(vi) Deviation from approved standards of calibration to be investigated appropriately (since the last successful calibration).

D. Computerized systems :

(i) GMP related computerized systems should be validated.

(ii) Installation Qualification (IQ) and Operation Qualification (OQ) for hardware and software must be established.

(iii) Commercially available qualified software if it is not validated at the time of installation, retrospective validation may be conducted and documented.

(iv) Software should have sufficient controls to prevent unauthorized access or change the data.

(v) Written SOP for operation and maintenance of computer system should be in place.

(vi) For critical data entry by manual should be checked by a second person.

(vii) Incidents which affect the reliability of records should be recorded and investigated.

(viii) Computerized system changes (hardware, software and critical components etc) should be according to documented change control procedure.

(ix) Back-up system with appropriate data protection should be established.

(x) Recording of data by a second source in addition to computer is acceptable to provide a back-up data source.

5.2.6 Documentation and Records

A. Documentation system and specifications :

(i) SOP for preparation. Review, approval and distribution of documents must be in place and it should be in paper or electronic form.

(ii) Issue, revisions, superseding and withdrawal of documents should be controlled.

(iii) SOP for maintenance of records with appropriate retention period should be established.

(iv) All production, control and distribution records should be maintained for atleast one year after the expiry date of the batch. For the APIs with retest dates, records must be stored for atleast 3 yrs after the batch is completely distributed.

(v) All the entries in the records should be orderly and signed. Correction to entries should be dated and signed and leave the original entry still readable.

(vi) Records can be either in microfilm or electronic forms. Hard copy should be readily available.

(vii) Specifications should be documented for raw materials, intermediates, APIs, labeling and packing materials, certain other materials such as process aids, gaskets etc should be documented with acceptance criteria.

(viii) Electronic signatures on documents are acceptable provided they are authenitic and secure.

B. Equipment cleaning and use record :

(i) Equipment cleaning record should contain Date / time/Product, Cleaned by/Checked by.

(ii) For dedicated equipment, individual equipment records may not be necessary. However, records of cleaning, maintenance and use may be part of batch record.

C. Records for RM, intermediates, API labeling and packing materials :

(i) Records for all materials must be in pace. Final decision regarding rejected RM, intermediates, API, labeling and packing materials must be documented.

(ii) Master labels must be maintained for comparison to issued labels.

D. Master production instruction (Master Production and Control Records) (MPCR) :

(i) Master production instructions for each intermediate and API should be prepared, dated and signed by one, independently checked, dated and signed by second person in the quality unit.

(ii) Master production instruction should include but not limited to :

(a) Name of the material and doc. Reference.

(b) Complete list of the materials and quality characteristics.

(c) Quantities of each material with identification.

(d) Production location and equipment used.

(e) Detailed production instructions like sequence of instructions, ranges of process parameters, sampling instructions, in-process controls and their acceptance criteria, time limits for completing, yield ranges.

(f) Cross references and precautions to be followed.

(g) Storage conditions to assure their suitability for use, including labeling and packing materials.

E. Batch Production and Control Records (BPCR) :

(i) Batch production records should include information relating to production, and control of each batch should be checked before issue to assure that it is correct version, legible and accurate reproduction of master production instructions. If BPCR is produced from the separate master document, the document should have reference to the current master production instruction.

(ii) BPCR should be numbered with a unique batch number, dated and signed.

(iii) Written procedure for investigating critical deviations or the failure of a batch intermediate or API to meet specifications.

(iv) Intermediate and APIs failing to meet established specifications should be identified as such and quarantined. Written procedure for re-process or rework should be established. The final disposition of rejected materials should be recorded.

(v) Completion of each significant step must include date and time, equipment used, specifications, weights, details of process deviations, Out of Specifications (OOS), results of critical process parameters, sampling, signature of the persons performing and checking each critical step in the operation, in-process results, yield particulars, description of label and packing operations, representative label, results of release testing etc.

F. Laboratory Control Records :

(i) Laboratory control records include complete data derived from all tests as per specifications and include.

(a) Description : Material name, B.No, date of sampling, quantity drawn, date the sample was received for testing.

(b) Reference to each test method used.

(c) Weight or measure of sample used for each test, cross-reference to the preparation and testing of laboratory enclosures.

(d) Raw data, spectra, charts enclosures.

(e) Record of calculations.

(f) Statement of the test results.

(g) Signature of the person, date and time.

(h) Signature of the reviewed person for accuracy, completeness and compliance with established standards.

(ii) Records should be maintained for

(a) any modifications to an established analytical method

(b) Calibration records.

(c) Stability data

(d) OOS investigations.

G. Batch Production Record Review :

(i) Written procedure must be established for review and approval of batch record, laboratory records, including packing and labeling, to determine compliance before the batch is released.

(ii) Critical steps results should be reviewed and approved by the quality units before the batch is released.

(iii) Deviations and OOS reports should be reviewed before the batch is released.

(iv) The quality units may delegate to the production units, the responsibility and authority for release of intermediates for in-house distribution.

5.2.7 Material Management

A. General Controls :

(i) Written SOP for receipt, identification, storage, handling, quarantine, sampling, testing, and approval or rejection of materials.

(ii) Evaluation of suppliers of critical materials.

(iii) Materials must be purchased from approved suppliers approved by Quality units and with agreed specifications.

(iv) For critical materials, manufacturer's name and address must be known.

(v) Change of the source of supply for critical material must be through change control decision.

B. Receipt and Quarantine :

(i) Before acceptance, materials should be examined for correct labeling, broken seals, container damage, evidence of tampering etc. materials should be held under quarantine until they have been sampled tested and released before use.

(ii) For bulk supply in non-dedicated containers, assurance of no cross contamination must be established by any of the following methods.

(a) Certificate of cleaning.

(b) Testing for trace impurities.

(c) Audit of the suppliers.

(iii) Identification system for status of materials must be in good order.

C. Sampling and testing of materials :

(i) For critical/active materials, at least one identification test of each batch materials must be established, supplier's Certificate of Analysis (COA) may be used to release the materials provided the manufacturer has a system to evaluate suppliers.

(ii) Processing aids, hazardous or toxic materials and special materials can be accepted based on supplier's COA.

(iii) Sampling of materials must be as per sampling plan with ensure representative sample and sufficient quantity for analysis.

(iv) The sampled containers must be properly identified and carefully re-closed after analysis.

D. Storage :

(i) Materials should be stored and handled to prevent degradation, contamination and cross-contamination.

(ii) Materials should be stored under set storage conditions and First - in - First - out (FIFO) should be followed for distribution.

(iii) Rejected materials should be identified and controlled to prevent unauthorized use in manufacturing.

E. Re-evaluation :

(i) Materials should be re-evaluated as appropriate to determine their suitability for use.

5.2.8 Production and in – Process Controls

A. Production operation :

(i) Weighing and measuring devices should be of suitable accuracy for the intended use.

(ii) Critical weights and measuring should be checked by production personnel.

(iii) Critical activities should be supervised.

(iv) Actual yields should be compared with expected yield range. Expected yield ranges can be arrived based on previous laboratory data, pilot scale experiments or past manufacturing data. Deviations in yield in critical process steps should be investigated.

(v) The processing status should be indicted by appropriate documentation.

(vi) Reprocessed or reworked materials should be controlled to prevent unauthorized use.

B. Time limits :

(i) Time limits for operations documented should match with master formula instructions. Deviation should be documented and evaluated. Time limits for in-process measurement steps may be inappropriate because completion of reactions are determined by in process sampling and testing.

(ii) Intermediates must be stored under appropriate storage conditions before processing to assure their suitability for use.

C. In- Processing sampling and controls :

(i) Written procedures should be established to monitor the progress and performance of the processing. In- process controls and their acceptance criteria should be defined based on development report or historical data.

(ii) Less stringent in-process controls in early processing steps and tighter controls for final stage intermediates desirable.

(iii) Critical process controls, control points and methods should be approved by quality unit.

(iv) Critical process tests and results should be documented in the batch record.

(v) Documented sampling plans for in-process materials, intermediates and APIs should be based on scientifically sound sampling practices.

(vi) In-process sampling should be carried out using dedicated samplers and by following documented procedures to prevent cross-contaminations.

5.2.9 Packing and Labeling of APIS and Intermediates for Transport

A. General :

(i) Documented procedure must be established for :

(a) Receipt

(b) Identification

(c) Quarantine

(d) Sampling

(e) Examination and/or testing and release

(f) Handling of packing, and labeling materials

(ii) Packing and labeling materials must conform to specifications before release and use, or otherwise, reject.

(iii) Records for packing and labeling materials for each shipment must be in place.

B. Packing materials :

(i) Containers should be clean, should be protected against deterioration during usage and transportation.

(ii) Containers should not be reactive, additive or absorptive.

(iii) Documented cleaning procedure for re-used containers must be in place. Previous labels must be defaced.

C. Label issuance and control :

(i) Access to label storage area should be limited to authorized personnel.

(ii) Label reconciliation procedure must be in place. Discrepancies should be investigated by quality unit.

(iii) Obsolete, rejected and out-dated labels must be destroyed.

(iv) Printing devices used to print labels must be controlled.

(v) Printed labels issued for a batch should match with specifications included in Master production record.

(vi) Specimen label must be included in the batch record.

D. Packing and labeling operation :

(i) Documented procedure for use of packing and labeling materials must be in place.

(ii) Label storage must be in identified locations to prevent mix-ups.

(iii) Label should indicate batch details, expiry/re-test date and storage conditions. Expiry/re-test date should be indicated on the certificate of analysis.

(iv) Packing and labeling facilities inspection status should be documented in the batch record.

(v) Packing details must be documented in the packing record.

(vi) Tamper proof seals must be used to the containers. The recipient must be communicated of this information.

5.2.10 Storage and Distibution

A. Warehousing Procedures :

(i) Adequate space and facilities should be available for storage of materials. The appropriate and applicable storage conditions (Temp, humidity where necessary) should be maintained. Records should be maintained.

(ii) Identified storage facilities for quarantine, approved, rejected, recalled materials must be available.

B. Distribution Procedures :

(i) APIs should be released for distribution only after approval by quality unit. Quarantine APIs may be transferred to another unit under the company's control by authorization by quality unit with appropriate storage control and documentation.

(ii) Transportation of APIs must be proper without affecting the quality.

(iii) Transportation and storage conditions must be stated on the label.

(iv) The transport contractors must be educated of transport and storage conditions to be maintained.

(v) Appropriate documentation system must be in place to recall the products immediately if necessary.

5.2.11 Laboratory Control

A. General Controls

(i) The quality unit must be independent of production unit and should be equipped with adequate laboratory facilities.

(ii) Documented procedure to describe
   (a) Sampling
   (b) Testing
   (c) Approval or rejection of materials and
   (d) Recording and storage of laboratory data.

(iii) Laboratory records should adequately address all the details.

(iv) Specifications, test methods, sampling plans including changes must be maintained.

(v) Specifications derived/documented must be in accordance with accepted standards and consistent with the manufacturing process. The specifications should include control of the impurities and appropriate microbiological purity levels.

(vi) Any deviations of laboratory controls from established procedures must be documented and justified.

(vii) Any out-of-specification (OOS) result obtained must be investigated and documented according to the procedure. This procedure should deal with:
   - Analysis of data
   - Assessment of significance of the problem.
   - Allocation of tasks for corrective action.
   - Conclusions
   - Re sampling and/or retesting after OOS results.

(viii) Primary standards should be obtained for APIs. This chapter should include:
   (a) Source of primary standards.
   (b) Records for storage and use
   (c) Storage conditions as per supplier's recommendations.
   (d) Testing of primary standards. (No testing is required if obtained from an official recognized source and if stored as per supplier's recommendations).

(ix) Where a primary standard is necessary and if not available from an official recognized source, an "in-house primary standard" should be prepared and established. This standard should be prepared by independent synthesis or by further purification of existing production materials. Characterization studies must be carried out to establish fully the identity and purity. Records should be maintained of these testing.

(x) Secondary laboratory reference standards must be prepared, identified, tested, approved and stored. The suitability of each batch of secondary reference standards should be determined before use by comparing with a primary reference standard. Each batch of secondary reference standard should be requalified periodically as per the written protocol.

B. Testing of Intermediates and APIs :

(i) Each batch of intermediate and API must be tested for conformance with established specifications.

(ii) An impurity profile describing identified and unidentified impurities present in a typical batch produced by a specific controlled conditions process should be established for each API.

The impurity profile include :

(a) Identification of impurities.

(b) Organic impurities/side products/degradants

(c) Inorganic impurities/ process aids

(d) Solvents

(iii) The impurity profile should be compiled and compared at regular intervals against the impurity profile data submitted to the regulatory agencies and against historical data in order to detect changes to the API resulting with use and modifications in raw materials, equipment operating parameters or process.

(iv) Microbiological tests must be conducted on each batch of intermediate or API where necessary.

C. Validation of Analytical Procedure (5.2.12)

D. Certificates of Analysis (COA)

(i) Authentic COA must be issued for each batch of intermediate or API.

(ii) Material grade, batch number, date of release, expiry date must be mentioned on the label and COA. The applicable retest date must be indicated on the label and COA.

(iii) The COA should include all tests, including acceptance limits and numerical results.

(iv) COA must be dated and signed by authorized personal of quality unit and should contain manufacturers name, address and telephone number. The repacker or reprocessor where appropriate, the name, address and telephone number must be described and original manufacture's reference should be indicated.

(v) If a new COA is issued on behalf of reprocessor, the COA should indicate name, address and telephone number of the laboratory where testing was performed. Additionally, the copy of original manufacturer's COA to be attached.

E. Stability Monitoring of APIs :

(i) A documented procedure/ programme to maintain stability testing should include at least.

(a) Storage conditions.

(b) Stability characteristics

(c) Results

(d) Retest or expiry dates.

(ii) The test method used should be a stability indicative and should be validated.

(iii) Stability samples should be stored in containers to simulate market conditions. The containers used must be of the same material, which should be in smaller size.

(iv) Generally, the first three commercial batches should be placed on stability to confirm retest or expiry date.

(v) At least one batch per year should be added to the stability-monitoring program.

(vi) For short life APIs, testing frequencies must be increased. Monthly, for first three months, and at three months intervals after that.

F. Expiry and Retest dating :

(i) When retest or expiry date is assigned, support stability information must be available (support e.g. published data, test results).

(ii) For API, expiry or retest date should be based on stability studies data. A common practice is that use retest date not expiration date.

(iii) Preliminary expiry or retest date should be based on pilot scale batches if pilot batches employ same manufacturing process and quality of API must have same characteristics.

(iv) Always a representative sample must be taken for testing.

G. Reserve/Reiteration samples :

(i) Reserve samples must be maintained to evaluate the quality of batches at a later date if necessary. These samples must be for potential future evaluation and not for future stability testing.

(ii) Reserve samples should be retained for one year after the expiry date of the batch assigned by the manufacturer or 3 years after distribution of the batch, whichever is longer.

(iii) The reserve samples must be stored under conditions consistent with product label condition, in the same packing conditions. Sufficient quantity should be retained to conduct at least two full specification analysis.

5.2.12 Validation

A. Validation policy :

(i) Company's overall policy, intentions and approach for validation should include

(a) Production process

(b) Cleaning procedures

(c) Analytical methods

(d) Test procedures (in process controls)

(e) Computerized system

(f) Personnel for design, review, approval and documentation.

(ii) Identification of critical parameters during development stage, based on historical data and ranges for operation.

(iii) Validation of process should be extended to other operations critical to control the quality and purity of API.

B. Validation Documentation :

(i) Written validation protocol to specify the validation process. Additionally, this should be reviewed and approved by quality unit.

(ii) The validation protocol should specify the type of validation to be carried out and also should indicate critical process steps and acceptance criteria. Also should include the number of runs to be considered.

(iii) Validation report should contain

(a) Cross reference to the validation protocol.

(b) Summary of results.

(c) Deviations noticed.

(d) Conclusions.

(e) Recommendations to correct deficiencies

(iv) Any changes proposed to be carried out to the plan defined in the validation protocol should be documented with justification.

C. Qualification

(i) Before starting processes validation activities, appropriate equipment and ancillary systems qualifications should be completed.

Qualifications should include

(a) ***Design qualification (DQ) :*** Documented verification of proposed design facilities, equipment or system is suitable for the intended purpose.

(b) ***Installation qualification (IQ) :*** Documented verification that the equipment or system as installed comply with the design parameters and manufacturer's recommendations.

(c) ***Operational qualification (OQ) :*** Documented verification that the equipment or system as installed performs as intended throughout the anticipated operating ranges.

(d) ***Performance qualification (PQ) :*** Documented verification that the equipment or system as installed can perform effectively and reproducible based on the approved process method and specification.

D. Approaches to process validation :

(i) Process validation (PV) is the documented evidences that the process (Operated within established parameter) can perform effectively and reproducible to produce either intermediate or API meeting its predetermined specifications and attributes.

(ii) There are three approaches to process validation. Prospective validation is the preferred approach.

(iii) *Prospective validation :* This should be completed on the API process before the commercial distribution of the final product.

(iv) *Concurrent validation :* This should be conducted when the data from replicate production runs are not available because only a limited number of API batches have been produced or API batches produced in frequently or API batches are produced by a validated process that has been modified prior to completion of concurrent validation, batches may be released and used in the final drug product for commercial distribution based on thorough monitoring and testing of API batches.

(v) *Retrospective process validation :* Can be conducted for a well established process without any significant changes to API quality due to change in

(a) Raw materials

(b) Equipment

(c) Systems

(d) Facilities

(e) Production process

This approach can be used where :

(a) Critical quality attributes and critical process parameters have been identified.

(b) In process acceptance criteria must be established.

(c) No significant process/ product failure attributable to causes other than operator error or equipment failure unrelated to equipment suitability.

(d) Impurity profiles must be established.

(e) Batches selected must be representative of all batches made during review period including failed batches and include sufficient number to demonstrate process consistency. Additional testing of retained samples may be needed for additional dated/information.

E. Process Validation Program :

(i) The number of process runs required for validation depends on the complexity of the process or magnitude of the process change being considered.

For Prospective and Concurrent validation, three consecutive successful production batches.

For retrospective validation, ten to thirty consecutive batches. Fewer batches may be examined if justified.

(ii) Critical process parameters should be controlled and monitored during process validation studies. Process parameters unrelated to quality need not be included.

(iii) Process validation should confirm that the impurity profile of each API is within the established limits.

F. Periodic Review of Validated Systems :

(i) Systems and process should be periodically evaluated to verify that they are under control. When no significant changes have been made to system or process, a quality review to evidence that the system or process will consistently produce the product meeting specifications will meet the need for revalidation.

G. Cleaning Validation :

(i) Cleaning procedures should normally be validated

Cleaning validation is required where the incidental carryover of materials poses the greatest risk to API quality.

Early production stages need not be validated where residues are removed by subsequent purification steps.

(ii) If various intermediates or APIs are manufactured in the same equipment and the equipment is cleaned by the same process, a representative intermediate or API may be selected for cleaning validation.

The selection depends upon the solubility and difficulty of cleaning. The residue limits are based on potency, toxicity and stability.

(iii) Cleaning validation protocol should include

(a) Equipment to be cleaned

(b) Procedure

(c) Materials used

(d) Acceptable cleaning levels

(e) Parameters to be monitored and controlled

(f) Analytical method

(g) Samples collection, labeling and type of samples

(iv) Sampling techniques should include

(a) Swabbing

(b) Rinsing

(c) Or any alternative method

(d) To detect both insoluble and soluble residues.

(e) The sampling method should be capable of quantitatively measure levels of residues remaining on the equipment surfaces after cleaning.

(f) Swab sampling may be impractical when product contact surfaces are not easily accessible due to equipment design (ex : transfer pipes, inner surfaces of hoses, reactor, tanks with small ports, micronizers etc.)

(v) The testing method should be validated. The detection limit of the method should be sufficiently sensitive to detect the established acceptable level of residue.

The cleaning method should indicate the recovery level. Residue limits should be practical, achievable and verifiable.

(vi) Equipment cleaning studies should address microbiological and endotoxins examination.

(vii) Cleaning procedures should be monitored at appropriate intervals after validation to ensure that these procedures are effective. Cleaning may be monitored by analytical testing and visual examination wherever feasible.

H. Validation of analytical methods :

(i) Analytical methods should be validated under the method employed is included in the current edition of an official pharmacoepia.

(ii) Method validation should include all the characteristics as per ICH guidelines on validation of analytical methods.

(iii) The appropriate qualification of analytical equipment should be considered before the method validation studies.

(iv) Analytical records should be maintained. Modification of method should produce the results that are as accurate and reliable as the established method.

5.2.13 Change Control

(i) A formal change control system should be established to evaluate all the changes that may affect the production and control of the intermediates or APIs.

(ii) Written procedure should be formalised to address identification, documentation, review and approval of changes in

(a) Raw materials

(b) Specifications

(c) Test methods

(d) Facilities

(e) Support systems

(f) Equipment and computer hardware

(g) Processing steps

(h) Labeling and packaging materials

(i) Computer software

(iii) GMP related changes should be drafted, by the appropriate units and reviewed and approved by the Quality units.

(iv) The potential impact of the proposed changes should be evaluated and justification should be documented. Changes may be classified as 'Minor' or 'Major' depending on the nature of changes and based on the effects that these changes may impact on the process and Quality. Validation may need to be carried out depending on the justification of change.

(v) While implementing the approved changes, ensure that all documents affected by the changes are reviewed and approved.

(vi) After the change has been implemented, evaluate the first few batches produced or tested under the change.

(vii) The batches may be added to the stability monitoring programme for accelerated stability and evaluate retest or expiry dates wherever necessary and essential.

(viii) Where the change can have impact on the quality of the API, dosage from manufactures, customs and regulatory authorities should be notified of the changes made from the established process.

5.2.14 Rejection and Re-Use of Materials

A. Rejection :

(a) Intermediate and APIs failing to meet established specifications should be identified and quarantined. The rejected materials should be either reprocessed or removed. The disposition of the rejected materials should be recorded.

B. Reprocessing :

(i) The materials, which do not conform to, established specifications, back into the process and reprocessing by repeating a step, which is a part of the established manufacturing process is also acceptable.

Ex : crystallization, physical manipulation, distillation, filtration, milling etc.

Additionally, if such reprocessing is used for majority of batches, such reprocessing should be included as a part of standard batch manufacturing process.

(ii) Continuation of an In-process control step, which is due to incompletion of reaction, is considered to be part of the normal process and should not be considered to be reprocessing.

(iii) Introducing unreacted materials back into the process and repeating a chemical reaction is considered to be reprocessing unless it is a part of the established process.

C. Reworking :

(i) Investigation of non-conformed materials, which do not conform to standard specifications, must be evaluated far before recommending for rework.

(ii) Reworked batches must be subjected to appropriate evaluation and testing. Also should be subjected for stability studies.

Equivalence statement documentation to show that reworked material is equivalent to the standard material must be established. Concurrent validation for reworked procedures, which include a protocol, which describes the rework procedure, how it will be carried out and the expected results. If only one batch is to be considered, interim report can be written and the batch is released if it is found acceptable.

(iii) Impurity profile of each reworked batch against batches manufactured by an established process, the procedure to be documented. Additional testing using additional methods must be established to evaluate such materials where routine analytical methods are found inadequate.

D. Recovery of Materials and Solvents :

(i) Established standard procedures to recover the reactants, intermediates and APIs from mother liquors or filtrates and ensure the recovered materials meet established specifications.

(ii) Solvents may be recovered and reused either in the same process or different processes provided the recovered materials meet appropriate specifications.

(iii) Fresh and recovered solvents may be combined after adequate testing and suitability of the materials in the process.

(iv) The use of recovered solvents, recovered materials, and mother liquors should be adequately documented.

E. Returns :

(i) Returned intermediates or APIs should be identified and quarantined.

(ii) If the condition of the returned containers casts doubt on the quality, the returned materials must be either reprocessed or recovered or destroyed as appropriate.

(iii) Records should be maintained, the documentation should include

(a) Name and address of the consignee

(b) Name of the material

(c) Batch number and quantity

(d) Reason for return

(e) Use of disposal and materials.

5.2.15 Complaints and Recalls

(i) Written procedure must be established for the receipt and investigation of the Quality complaints received either in writing or orally.

(ii) Complaint record should include.

(a) Name and address of complainant.

(b) Name and telephone number of person submitting the complaint.

(c) Nature of complaint.

(d) Date of receipt of complaint.

(e) Action taken.

(f) Response to the originator of complaint.

(g) Final decision.

(iii) Records should be retained to evaluate trends and for initiating necessary corrective action.

(iv) Written procedure should be established to recall the materials

(v) The recall procedure should be defined to address

(a) Who should be involved in evaluating the information

(b) How a recall should be initiated

(c) Who should be informed about the recall

(d) How a recalled material should be tested

(vi) In the event of potential life-threatening situation, local, national and International authorities should be informed and their advice sought.

5.2.16 Contract Manufacturers (Including Laboratories)

(i) All the contract manufacturers should comply with the GMP(s) with specific reference for identification of materials and to present cross-contamination.

(ii) Contract Manufacturers should be evaluated by the contract giver to GMP compliance of specific operations occurring at the contract sites.

(iii) There should be a written and approved contract between contract giver and the contract acceptor, which defines in detail the GMP, and quality related matters.

(iv) The contract should permit the contract giver to audit the contract acceptor's facility for compliance with GMPs.

(v) The contract acceptor should not pass to a third party any of the work entrusted to him without the contract giver's prior evaluation and approval of the third party facilities

(vi) Manufacturing and analytical records should be made available at the site.

(vii) Changes in the process, equipment, test methods, specifications and any other contractual requirements should not be made unless the contract giver approves the changes.

5.2.17 Agents, Brokers, Distributors, Re-packers and Re-labelers

A. Applicability :

(i) Applicable to both API and intermediates.

(ii) Applies to any party other than original manufacturer. The agency may be a Trader, or possess the material, handle, re-pack, re-label, manipulate or stored.

(iii) All the agencies mentioned above must comply with GMPs.

B. Tractability of Distributed APIs :

(i) Agents, Brokers, Distributors, Re-packers, Re-labelers should maintain Complete tractability of material they distribute.

Documents should be retained and must include

(a) Identity of original manufacturer

(b) Address of original manufacturer

(c) Purchase orders

(d) Bills of lading (transportation documentation)
(e) Receipt documents
(f) Name of the API
(g) Manufacturer's batch number
(h) Transportation and distribution records
(i) COA of original manufacturer
(j) Date of manufacture and expiry or retest date

C. Quality Management :

All agents, brokers, distributors, re-packers or re-labelers should establish, document and implement an effective QMS.

D. Re-packing, Re-labeling and Holding of APIs.

(i) Re-packing, Re-labeling and holding of APIs should be performed under appropriate GMP controls to avoid mix-ups and loss of identity.

(ii) Re-packing should be conducted under appropriate environmental conditions to avoid contamination and cross-contamination.

E. Stability :

(i) Stability studies to justify the assigned expiration or retest dates should be conducted if the APIs are re-packed in a different type of container than that used by the API manufacturer.

F. Transfer of Information :

(i) Agents, Brokers, Distributors, Re-packers or Re-labelers should transfer all Quality related information received from API manufacturer to the customer and from the customer to the API manufacturer.

(ii) The above agencies that supply the API to the customer should provide the name of the API manufacturer and the batch numbers supplied.

(iii) The agent should provide the identity of the original API manufacturer to regulatory authorities upon request. The original manufacturer may respond directly with the regulatory authorities wherever required.

(iv) COA should be included along with the consignment.

G. Handling of Complaints and Recalls :

(i) The agencies listed above must maintain records of complaints and recalls, which come to their attention.

(ii) If the situation warrants, the agencies should review the complaint with the original manufacturer and investigation should be initiated.

(iii) The agency should maintain the response of the complaint from the manufacturer.

H. Handling of Returns :

(i) The agencies listed above should maintain documentation for returned goods/APIs.

5.2.18 Specific Guidance for APIs Manufacturer by Cell Culture/Fermentation

A. General :

(i) This section refers to APIs or intermediates manufactured by cell culture or fermentation. In general, the degree of control for biotech process is greater than those used in classical fermentation process.

(ii) Production of APIs or intermediates from cell culture or fermentation involves biological process, extraction and purification of materials from living organisms. The control of bio-burden, viral contamination, and/or endotoxins during manufacturing and monitoring the process at appropriate stages may be necessary.

(iii) Appropriate process controls at all stages of manufacture to protect the quality are necessary. The controls start from the point at which a vial of cell bank is retrieved from the laboratory for use in the manufacturing.

(iv) Appropriate environmental controls and equipments should be used. Frequency of environmental monitoring is necessary.

(v) The process controls should include

(a) Preservation of mother culture

(b) Maintenance of working culture

(c) Inoculation and expansion of the culture

(d) Control of critical operating parameters during fermentation.

(e) Monitoring the cell growth process, viability and productivity.

(f) Harvest and purification procedures to remove cellular debris and protecting the intermediate from contamination and particularly microbiological nature contamination.

(g) Bio-burden and endotoxin levels should be monitored at appropriate stages of production.

(h) Viral safety concerns should be followed ass per ICH Q5A: Quality of Bio-technological products.

(vi) For biotech products, validation of the removal of media components, host cell proteins, other process-related impurities, product related impurities and contaminants may be necessary.

B. Cell bank maintenance and Record keeping :

(i) Access to cell bank should be limited to authorized personnel.

(ii) Cell bank should be maintained under designed storage conditions to maintain viability and to prevent contamination

(iii) Records for use of cell vials and storage conditions should be maintained.

(iv) Cell banks should be periodically monitored to determine the suitability of use. The number of passages should be decided and defined.

(v) Characterization of cell substances : ICHQ5D

C. Cell Culture/Fermentation :

(i) Closed or contained systems should be used to permit the aseptic addition of cell substrates, media buffers and gases etc. inoculation of media and transfer or addition for media buffers should be as per designated procedures to minimize contamination.

(ii) Bio-safety cabinet should be maintained under controlled environmental conditions.

(iii) Personnel should be properly gowned and special precautions to be taken while handling the cultures.

(iv) Critical operating parameters like temperature, PH, agitation rates, addition of gases; pressure should be monitored to ensure consistency of the process. Cell growth, viability and productivity should be monitored.

(v) Cell culture and fermentation equipment should be cleaned and sterilized after use.

(vi) Culture media should be sterilized before use to protect the quality of API.

(vii) Procedure should be in place to detect contamination and determine the course of action to be taken. Procedure for the determination of foreign organisms during fermentation process should be in place, which also should deal with the effect of such organisms on the product quality.

(viii) Records of contamination events should be maintained.

(ix) Multi-product equipments require additional cleaning and testing between product campaigns is necessary to minimize cross-contamination.

D. Harvesting, Isolation and Purification :

(i) Harvesting to remove the cells from media and the areas to minimize the contamination is important.

(ii) Harvesting and purification procedures should deal with the removal of inactive organisms, cell debris etc.

(iii) All equipment should be properly cleaned and sanitized after used.

(iv) Suitable environmental conditions during production should be maintained and quality use of HEPA filtered air is recommended.

(v) Additional purification controls if required in the process, should be highlighted.

E. Viral Removal/Inactivation Steps :

(i) Ref : ICH Q5A

(ii) Critical process steps (viral removal/inactivation) should be validated.

(iii) Open processing should be performed in separate areas with separate air handling units.

(iv) Preferably dedicated equipment should be used in the purification steps.

5.2.19 API for Use in Clinical Trials

A. General:

(i) Specific guidance for clinical trials as appropriate should be considered.

(ii) Steps to be followed from pre-clinical stages. By the time the drug development reaches the stage of final clinical trails, manufacturer should ensure that APIs are manufactured in suitable facilities, using appropriate production and controlled procedures to ensure the quality of API.

B. Quality :

(i) GMP controls should be applied in the production.

(ii) Quality Unit is independent of production.

(iii) testing equipment can be common.

(iv) Quality parameters at all stages should be in place.

(v) Process and quality problems should be evaluated.

(vi) Labeling should be appropriate.

C. Equipment and Facilities :

(i) During all stages of clinical development, procedures should be in place to ensure equipment calibration, cleanliness and use of suitable equipment.

(ii) The facilities should ensure that materials are handled in such a manner to minimize the risk of contamination and cross-contamination.

D. Control of Raw Materials :

(i) Raw materials should be appropriately controlled. For hazardous materials, supplier's analysis should suffice.

(ii) In some cases, suitability of raw materials may be determined by performance resting rather than analytical testing alone.

E. Production :

(i) The production details should be documented in laboratory note books, batch records etc. These records include details of production materials, equipment, processing and specific observations.

F. Validation :

(i) Process validation may be inappropriate during clinical API production.

(ii) Process validation should be conducted on commercial plant batches or pilot-scale batches. (Section XII)

G. Changes :

(i) Although changes are expected during clinical development, changes made during production, test procedures or specifications should be recorded.

H. Laboratory Controls :

(i) All testing carried out to evaluate a batch of API for clinical trails should be scientifically sound, the methods may not be fully validated.

(ii) Reserve samples of sufficient quantity of all batches should be maintained.

(iii) Expiry or retest periods though essential for APIs (section XI.F), do not apply in early stages of clinical trial materials.

I. Documentation :

(i) Product and process development information from laboratory to manufacture should be documented.

(ii) The development and implementation of analytical methods to support the release of API should be documented.

(iii) Production and control records should be retained for appropriate length of time.

5.2.20 Glossary

Active Pharmaceutical Ingredient (API) (drug substance) :

Any substance or mixture of substance intended to be used in the manufacture of a drug (medicinal) product and that when used in the production of a drug becomes an active ingredient of the drug product. Such substances are intended to furnish pharmacological activity or other direct effect in the diagnosis, cure, mitigation, treatment or prevention of disease or to affect the structure and function of the body.

API Starting material :

A material used in the production of an API, which is itself or is incorporated as a significant structural fragment into the structure of the API. An API starting material may be an article of commerce, a material of purchase from one or more suppliers under contract or commercial agreement, or it may be produced in-house. API starting materials are normally of defined chemical properties and structure.

Batch (or Lot) :

A specific quantity of material produced in a process or series of processes so that it is expected to be homogenous within specified limits. In the case of continuous production a batch may correspond to a defined fraction of the production. The batch size may be defined either by a fixed quantity or their amount produced in a fixed time interval.

Batch number or Lot number :

A unique combination of numbers, letters, and or symbols which identifies a batch and from which the production and distribution history can be determined.

Bio-burden :

The level and type (e.g. objectionable or not) of microorganisms which may be present in raw materials, API starting materials, intermediates or APIs. Bio-burden should not be considered contamination unless the levels have been exceeded or defined objectionable organisms have been detected.

Calibration :

The demonstration that a particular instrument or device produces results within specified limits by comparison with those produced by a reference or traceable standard over an appropriate range of measurements.

Computer system :

A group of hardware components and associated software, designed and assembled to perform a specific function or group of function.

Computerized system :

A process or operation integrated with a computer system.

Contamination :

The undesired introduction of impurities of a chemical or microbiological nature, or of foreign matter, into or onto a raw material, intermediate, or API during production, sampling, packing or repackaging, storage or transport.

Contract manufacturer :

A company holding an agreement requires the performance of some aspect of API manufacturing.

Critical :

A process step, process condition, test requirement or other relevant parameter or items that must be controlled within predetermined criteria to ensure that the API meets its specifications.

Cross-contamination :

Contamination of a material or a product with another material or product.

Drug (Medicinal) product :

The dosage form in the final immediate packing intended for marketing

Expiry/Expiration date :

The date placed on the container/label of an API designated the time during which the API is expected to remain with in established shelf life specifications if stored under defined conditions, and after which it should not be used.

Impurity :

Any component present in the intermediate or API that is not the desired entity.

Impurity profile :

A description of the identified and unidentified impurities present in an API.

In-process control also called process control :

Checks performed during production in order to monitor and if necessary to adjust the process and/ or to ensure that the intermediate or API conforms to its specification.

Intermediate :

A material produced during steps of the processing of an API which must undergo further molecular change or purification before it becomes an API. Intermediates may or may not be isolated.

Manufacture :

All operations of receipt of materials, production, packing, re-packing, labeling, re-labeling, quality control, release, storage and distribution of API and related controls.

Material :

A general term used to denote raw materials (starting materials, reagents, solvents) process aids, intermediates, APIs and packing and labeling materials.

Mother liquor :

The residual liquid remains after the crystallization or isolation processes. Mother liquor may contain unreacted materials, intermediates, levels of the API and/ or impurities. It may be used for further processing.

Packing material :

Any material intended to protect an intermediate or API during storage and transport.

Procedure :

A documented description of the operations to be performed, the precaution to be taken and measures to be applied directly or indirectly related to the manufacture of an intermediate or API.

Process aids :

Material excluding solvents used as aid in the manufacture of an intermediate or API which themselves do not participate in a chemical or biological reaction (e.g. filter aid, activated carbon etc).

Production :

All operations involved in the preparation of an API, from receipt of materials, through processing and packing, to its completion as a finished API.

Qualification :

Action of proving and documenting that equipment or ancillary systems are properly work correctly and actually lead to the expected results. Qualification is part of validation, but the individual qualification steps alone do not constitute process validation.

Quality assurance (QA) :

The sum total of the organized arrangements made with the object of ensuring that all APIs are of the quality required for their intended use and that quality system's are maintained.

Quality control (QC) :

Checking or testing those specifications are met.

Quality unit :

An organizational unit independent of production, which fulfills both quality assurance and quality control responsibilities. This may be in the form of separate QA and QC units, a single individual (or group), depending upon the size and structure of the organization

Quarantine :

The status of material isolated physically or by other effective means pending a decision on their subsequent approval or rejection.

Raw material :

A general term used to denote starting materials, reagents, and solvents intended for use in the production of intermediate or APIs.

Reference standard, primary :

A substance that has been shown by an extensive set of analytical tests to be authentic material, which should be of high purity. This standard may be obtained from an officially recognized source or may be prepared by an independent synthesis or further purification of existing production material.

Reference standard, secondary :

A substance of established quality and purity, as shown by comparison to a primary reference standard used as a reference standard for routine laboratory analysis.

Reprocessing :

Introducing an intermediate or API, including that which does not conform to standard or specifications, back into the process and repeating a crystallization step or other appropriate chemical or physical manipulation steps. (Eg; distillation, filtration, chromatography, milling etc) that are part of the established manufacturing process

Continuation of a chemical reaction after the in-process control test shows the reaction to be incomplete is considered to be part of the normal process and not reprocessing.

Retest date :

The date when a material should be re-examined to ensure that it is still suitable for use.

Reworking :

Subjecting an intermediate or API that does not conform to standards or specifications, to one or more processing steps that are different from the established manufacturing process so that its quality may be made acceptable (e.g.. re-crystallizing with a different solvent)

Signature (signed) :

See definition of signed

Signed (signature) :

The record of who performed a particular action or review. This record may be an initial, full handwritten signature, personal seal, or authenticated and secure electronic signature.

Solvent :

An inorganic or organic liquid used as a vehicle for the preparation of solutions or suspensions in the manufacture of an intermediate or API.

Specification :

A list of tests, references to analytical procedures, and appropriate acceptance criteria that are numerical limits, ranges or other criteria for the test described. It establishes the set of criteria to which a material should conform to be considered acceptable for its intended use. "Conformance to specification" means that the material, when tested according to the listed analytical procedures, will meet the listed acceptance criteria.

Validation :

A documented program that provides a high degree of assurance that a specific process, method or system will consistently produce a result meeting predetermined acceptance criteria.

Validation protocol :

A written plan stating how validation will be conducted and defining acceptance criteria. For example, the protocol for a manufacturing process identities, processing equipment, critical process parameters/ operating ranges, product characteristics, sampling, and test data to be collected, number of validation runs, and acceptable test results.

Yield, expected :

The quantity of material or the percentage of theoretical yield anticipated at any appropriate phase of production based on previous laboratory, pilot scale, or manufacturing data.

Yield, theoretical :

The quantity that would be produced at any appropriate phase of production, based upon the quantity of material to be used, in the absence of any loss or error in actual production.

5.3 Good Clinical Practices

- The guidelines on good clinical practice (GCP) for trials on pharmaceutical products are given below.
- To assure consistency between and within batches of the investigational product and thus assure the reliability of clinical trials.
- To assure consistency between the investigational product and the future commercial product and therefore the relevance of the clinical trial to the efficacy and safety of the marketed product.
- To protect subjects of clinical trials from poor-quality products resulting from manufacturing errors (omission of critical steps such as sterilization, contamination and cross-contamination, mix-ups, wrong labelling, etc.), or from starting materials and components of inadequate quality.
- To document all changes in the manufacturing process.

In this context, the selection of an appropriate dosage for clinical trials is important: While it is accepted that in early trials the dosage form may be very different from the anticipated final formulation (e.g. a capsule instead of a tablet), in the pivotal Phase III studies it should be similar to the projected commercial presentation otherwise these trials will not necessarily prove that the marketed product is both efficacious and safe.

If there are significant differences between the clinical and commercial dosage forms, data should be submitted to the registration authorities to demonstrate that the final dosage form is equivalent, in terms of bio avail ability and stability, to that used in the clinical trials. Final manufacturing methods must be revalidated following changes in processes, scaling up, transfer to other manufacturing sites, etc.

Glossary

The definitions given below apply to the terms used in these guidelines. They may have different meanings in other contexts.

Clinical trial

Any systematic study on pharmaceutical products in-human subjects, whether in patients or other volunteers, in order to discover or verify the effects of, and/or identify any adverse reaction to, investigational products, and/or to study the absorption, distribution, metabolism and excretion of the products with' the object of ascertaining their efficacy and safety.

Clinical trials are generally divided into Phases I-IV. It is not possible to draw clear distinctions between these phases, and different opinions about details and methodology do exist. However, the individual phases, based on their purposes as related to the clinical development of pharmaceutical products, can be briefly defined as follows :

Pharmaceutical product

For the purpose of this Annex, this term is defined in the same way as in the. WHO guidelines on GCP (3), i.e. as any substance or combination of substances which has a therapeutic, prophylactic or diagnostic purpose, or is intended to modify physiological functions, and is presented in a dosage form suitable for administration to humans.

Product specification filers(s)

Reference file(s) containing all the information necessary to draft the detailed written instructions on processing, packaging; labelling, quality control testing batch release, storage conditions and shipping.

Protocol

A document, which gives the background, rationale and objectives of the trial and describes its design, methodology and organization, including statistical considerations, and the conditions under which it is to be performed and managed. It should be dated and signed by the investigator/institution involved and the sponsor, and can, in addition, function as a contract.

Shipping/dispatch

The assembly, packing for shipment, and sending of ordered-medicinal products for clinical trials.

Sponsor

An individual, company, institution or organization which takes responsibility for the initiation, management and/or financing of a clinical trial. When an investigator independently initiates and takes full responsibility for a trial, the investigator then also assumes the role of the sponsor.

Good pharmacy practice

The practice of pharmacy aimed at providing and promoting the best use of drugs and other health care services and products, by patients and members of the public. It requires that the welfare of the patient is the pharmacist's prime concern at all times.

Over-the-counter drugs

These are drugs that can be sold from licensed dealers without professional supervision and without prescriptions. These drugs are suitable for self medication for minor diseases and symptoms.

Pharmacist

A pharmacist is a holder of a degree or diploma in pharmacy from a recognized higher institution of learning and is registered or licensed to practise pharmacy.

Pharmacy-only drugs

These are drugs authorized to be sold only in licensed pharmacies under the supervision of licensed and registered pharmacists; they may be sold without a prescription.

Phase I : These are the first trials of a new active ingredient or new formulations in humans, often carried out in healthy volunteers. Their purpose is to make a preliminary evaluation of safety, and an initial pharmacokinetic / pharmacodynamic profile of the active ingredient.

Phase II : The purpose of these therapeutic pilot studies is to determine activity and to assess the short-term safety of the active ingredient in patients suffering from a disease or condition for which it is intended. The trials are performed in a limited number of subjects and are often, at a later stage, of a comparative (e.g. placebo-controlled) design. This phase is also concerned with the determination of appropriate dose ranges/regimens and (if possible) the clarification of dose-response relationships in order to provide an optimal background for the design of extensive therapeutic trials.

Phase III : This phase involves trials in large (and possibly varied) patient groups for the purpose of determining the short- and long-term safety-efficacy balance -of formulation(s) of the active ingredient, and assessing its overall and relative therapeutic value. The pattern and profile of any frequent adverse reactions must be investigated, and special features o/the product must be explored (e.g. clinically relevant drug interactions, factors leading to differences in effect, such as age). The trials should preferably be randomized double blind, but other designs may be acceptable, e.g. long-term safety studies. In general, the conditions under which the trials ate cond4cted should be as close as possible to the normal conditions of use.

Phase IV : In this phase studies are performed after the pharmaceutical product has been marketed. They are based on the product characteristics on which the marketing authorization was granted and normally take the form of post-marketing surveillance, and assessment of therapeutic value or treatment strategies. Although methods may differ, the same scientific and ethical standards should apply to Phase IV studies as are applied in remarketing studies. After li product has been placed on the market, clinical trials designed to explote new indications, new methods of administration or new combirtatiollS, etc., are normally regarded as trials of new pharmaceutical products.

Investigational product

Any pharmaceutical product (new product or reference product) or placebo being tested or used as a reference in a clinical trial.

Investigator

The person responsible for the trial and for protecting the rights, health and welfare of the subjects in the trial. The investigator must be an appropriately qualified person legally allowed to practice medicine/ dentistry.

Monitor

A person appointed by, and responsible to, the/sponsor for monitoring and reporting the progress of the trial and for the verification of data.

Order

An instruction to process, package and/or ship a certain number of units of an investigational product.

Poison

A preparation or substance defined by a national drug law as a poison.

Prescription-only drugs

These are drugs supplied only in licensed pharmacies on the presentation of signed prescriptions issued by a licensed arid registered medical practitioner, licensed and/or registered dentist (for dental treatment only), and/or licensed and/or registered veterinarian (for animal treatment only), and the supply and dispensing of these drugs must be carried out by a pharmacist or under the supervision of a pharmacist. Prescription drugs are further subdivided into controlled drugs (narcotic drugs and psychotropic substances) and non-controlled drugs.

Product recall

Product recall is a process for withdrawing or removing a pharmaceutical product from the pharmaceutical distribution chain because of defects in the product or complaints of serious adverse reactions to the product. The recall might be initiated by the manufacturer/importer/distributor or a responsible agency.

Prohibited drugs

These are drugs with toxicity or side-effects that outweigh their therapeutic usefulness, so that public health and welfare are protected by prohibiting their production, manufacture, export; import, trade, distribution, supply, possession or use, except in amounts required for medical and scientific research. Prohibited drugs are normally determined by me national or supranational registration licensing authority.

Quality assurance

Quality assurance is a wide-ranging concept covering all matters that individually or collectively influence the quality of a product. It is the totality of the arrangements made with the object of ensuring that pharmaceutical products are of the quality required for their intended use.

Quality control

Quality control covers all measures taken, including the setting of specifications, sampling, testing and analytical clearance, to ensure that raw materials, intermediates, packaging materials and finished pharmaceutical products conform with established specifications for identity, strength, purity and other characteristics.

Unauthorized market (in some countries called parallel market)

The unauthorized market consists of wholesale establishments and retail outlets distributing or selling drugs without authorization from a competent.

Summary

The basic elements of Quality Management in a pharmaceutical Industries are :

Appropriate infrastructure and quality system, encompassing the organizational structure, procedures, processes, and resources;

Systematic actions necessary to ensure adequate confidence that a product (or service) will satisfy given requirements for quality. The totality of these actions are termed as "quality assurance".

"Quality Assurance" is a wide range concept covering all matters that individually or collectively influence the quality of a product. It is the totality of the arrangements made with the object of ensuring that pharmaceutical products are of required quality meeting their intended use",

With reference to pharmaceutical industry Quality Assurance will be done in which implementation of Good clinical practices (GCP), Good Manufacturing Practices (GMP), Good Laboratory Practices (GLP), exists. Thus Quality Assurance can be represented as,

Quality assurance = GCP + GMP + GLP other measures.

The manufacturer must assume responsibility for the quality of the pharmaceutical products to ensure that they are fit for their intended use, comply with the requirements of the marketing authorization and do not place patients at risk due to inadequate safety, quality, or efficacy.

Good Manufacturing practice is that part of quality assurance which ensures that products are consistently produced and controlled to the quality standards appropriate to their intended use and as required by the marketing authorization. GMP rules are directed primarily to diminishing the risks, inherent in any pharmaceutical production, that cannot be prevented completely through the testing of final products, such risks are essentially of two types: cross contamination (in particular by unexpected contaminants) and mix-ups (confusion) caused by false labels being put on containers. Under GMP:

All manufacturing processes are clearly defined, systematically reviewed in the light of experience, and shown to be capable of consistently manufacturing pharmaceutical products of the required quality that comply with their specifications;

Critical steps of manufacturing processes and any significant changes made to the processes are validated;

All necessary facilities are provided, including: Appropriately qualified and trained personnel; Adequate premises and space; Suitable equipment and services; Correct materials, containers, and labels; Approved procedures and instructions; Suitable storage and transport; and Adequate personnel, facilities, and equipment for in-process controls under the responsibility of the production management; Instructions and procedures, are written in clear and unambiguous language, specifically applicable to the facilities provided; Operators are trained to carry out procedures correctly:

Records are made (manually and/or by recording instruments) during manufacture to show that all the steps required by the defined procedures and instructions have in fact been taken and that the quantity and quality of the product are as expected; any significant deviations are fully recorded and investigated;

Records covering manufacture and distribution, which enable the complete history of a batch to be traced, are retained in a comprehensible and accessible form;

The proper storage and distribution of the products minimizes any risk to their quality;

A system is available to recall any batch of product from sale or supply;

Complaints about marketed products are examined; the causes of quality defects investigated, and appropriate measures taken in respect of the defective products and to prevent recurrence.

Questions

1. Define the following terms :
   (a) Inspection and testing
   (b) Quality Control
   (c) Total Quality Control
   (d) Quality Assurance
   (e) Continual improvement
2. What is the significance of Quality Assurance" in pharmaceutical Industry?

3. What are the Three the key functions of "Quality Management"?
4. What are the key contents to be described in a batch production record?
5. Discuss in detail the content of Master formula record? Why is it required?
6. Briefly describe the scope of GMP in a pharmaceutical industry and applicable departments?
7. Discuss in detail the activities of packing and labeling in Active Pharmaceutical substance manufacturing keeping regulatory perspective in view.
8. Discuss in detail the various activities needed to be carried out in pharmaceutical "Quality Control Laboratory".
9. What is the significance of conducting stability studies? Why is it required?
10. Define the term "Validation". Describe the contents of "Master Validation Plan".
11. What are the three types of carrying our process validation?
12. Discuss in detail the significant aspects of equipment cleaning and their importance.
13. Discuss the parameters to be studied or included in carrying our Assay Method validation.
14. Why change control system implementation is mandatory in Pharmaceutical industry?
15. How do you salvage a non-conforming product?
16. What do you mean by product recall? What are the implications involved in a product recall process?
17. Discuss in detail the responsibilities of an organisation to conduct an activity in a contract manufacturing facility.
18. What is the responsibility of traders and distributors in fulfilling their duties in the distribution activity of a pharmaceutical substance?

6

Statistical Quality Control

6.1 Introduction

Statistical quality control (SQC) is the use of carefully selected methods for improving product quality. It involves quick identification of any decline in quality during the initial stages of production and taking immediate corrective action instead of identifying defectives after the damage has been done. One of the methods used for identifying defects is sampling. "Why sampling, we may ask". The answer is that, 100% inspection of products is very time-consuming and expensive. And it has been scientifically proved that sampling almost always shows defects as well as 100 % inspection. Doing it right first time assumes great importance when it helps to avoid 100 % inspection.

6.1.1 Quality System at the Process Level – Statistical Process Control

It was found that control in the quality of the processes resulted in greater gains that by controlling the quality of the finished product. Controlling the quality of manufacturing processes not only improved product quality but also eliminated enormous wastage. Otherwise rejections are trapped only after the process is completed and at a stage when all the cost have already been incurred.

At the process level SQC (Statistical Quality Control) is introduced at every stage from design to dispatch. In other words quality control started mush earlier than the actual production. Training and motivation from a part of the quality control movement.

Statistical process control techniques help in controlling the manufacturing processes more effectively. These techniques monitor the manufacture process and control the quality of these processes. Manufacturers can stop the flow in the production line if and when it is required in case any anomalies are to be corrected or if they find that the process is deviating from norms.

In other words, SQC is a method to improve product quality, thereby limiting waste and rework. Naturally, production also increases.

The term 'statistical' method implies the collection of numerical data, which are tabulated, and summarized using prescribed statistical tools for the purpose of analysis and reporting.

As seen earlier, statistical analysis is done for a small sample of the products instead of 100 % inspection. This 'sample' on which the statistical analysis is done reveals the quality or decline in quality of the entire lot.

When statistical quality control is done on a scientific basis with careful sampling, then SQC helps in arriving at inferences of a similar nature of high validity within limited time and cost. Specific tools, graphs and charts are used for drawing relevant inferences from sample population.

6.2 Statistical Process Control

Statistical process control (SPC) was developed by W.Edward Deming, along with another expert, W.A.Shewhart (1). According to them any process or product that can be measured by its characteristics can be analysed using SPC. This is an extension of SQC to the processes instead of confining the statistical techniques to the products.

According to Deming, the American 'quality guru', quality in production can be achieved by:

(i) Identifying the cause of production problems

(ii) Carefully monitoring production to stop errors before too many products are made.

Deming divides the causes of problems into two categories – Common and Special causes. Common causes are systemic problems, common to the system and shared by many workers, machines and product types. Special causes are problems that relate to individual workers, machines or material shipments.

6.2.1 Statistical Process Control Tools

SPC can be applied by following a sequence of steps

At each stage, there are statistical tools that can be used. The steps and the corresponding tools are:

(i) Define the problem, identify primary causes, and prioritise areas to receive follow up attention (Pareto chart Fig. 6.1).

(ii) Determine the level of process control and the process capability of the primary possible process by the direct measurements from the operation (Control charts).

(iii) Identify potential causes of instability identified in the previous stage. (Fishbone diagram or Cause and effect diagram).

(iv) Quantify the relationship between the variables (process or product) of interest from the previous step and other process variables (Scatter diagram, and correlation studies).

(v) Confirm the effect of any process or equipment changes on process stability and capability (Control charts).

6.2.2 Pareto Chart

Pareto chart graphically depicts (Fig. 6.1.) the relationship between an identified problem and its causes. The idea is that, in general, 80 % of an effect can be attributed to 20 % (major) identifiable causes. It highlights the cause(s) that should be given the highest priority. You can see that this is the same concept as that of ABC analysis that we saw under Materials.

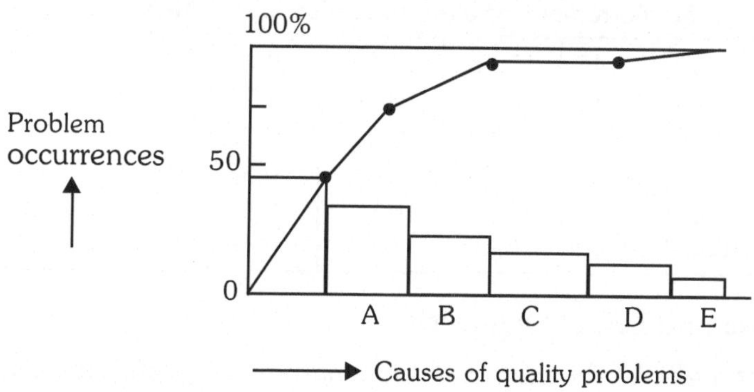

Figure 6.1 Pareto chart.

6.2.3 Control Charts

While measuring the characteristics of a process or product, we may observe variations in the values measured from the sample, due to various reasons.

For example, in a manufacturing set-up, the reasons could be :

- Machine set-up
- Tooling
- Temperature
- Voltage
- Compressed air pressure
- Operating errors
- Material quality
- Measuring equipment etc.

We can use Control charts to identify the extent of deviations that occur in the processes. Control charts are line graphs that record the number of defects. A control chart plots sampled data, representing process output, with respect to time, in a form that makes it easy to analyse whether the process is in control or out of control.

For the manufacturing processes the following are the observations of length measures of the samples taken at an interval of one hour (Table 6.1.). Five samples are taken every hour, and the mean length values are plotted on the control graph. It is found that length measurements vary in each sample.

Table 6.1 Cutting process – length measurements

Sigma = 0.02 mm

Time a.m.	Measurement of sample X mm					Mean	Range
6	10.50	10.47	10.48	10.47	10.48	10.48	0.03
7	10.48	10.50	10.52	10.49	10.51	10.50	0.04
8	10.51	10.52	10.52	10.53	10.52	10.52	0.02
9	10.53	10.54	10.53	10.54	10.56	10.54	0.03
10	10.49	10.50	10.48	10.53	10.50	10.50	0.05
11	10.47	10.45	10.46	10.47	10.45	10.46	0.02

6.2.4 Cause and Effect Diagram

The 'cause and effect', diagram as a tool can be very useful. It uses the four fundamental components of any process: machines, manpower, materials, and methods to ascertain the causes for out-of-control conditions.

These tools can be used for any type of industry. All employees are nowadays trained in using these tools. Once they have learnt to use these tools over a period of time, the usefulness of the tools will be reflected in the company's productivity.

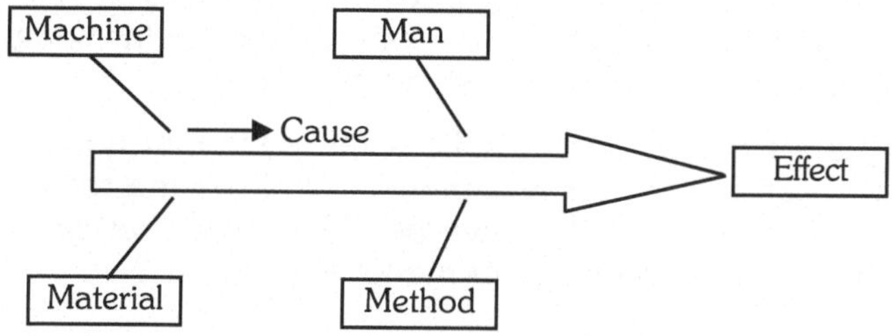

Figure 6.2 Cause and effect diagram.

6.2.5 Scatter Diagram

Using a combination of the above tools, once a set of possible causes and effects are identified, either from available data or through experimentation, a graph is drawn between a cause (X – axis) and an effect (Y – axis). For example, if it is found that a possible cause could be a machine going out of control over time, a scatter diagram could establish whether it is indeed true or not. In the following diagram the effect of a machine producing more defectives after each service is becoming apparent.

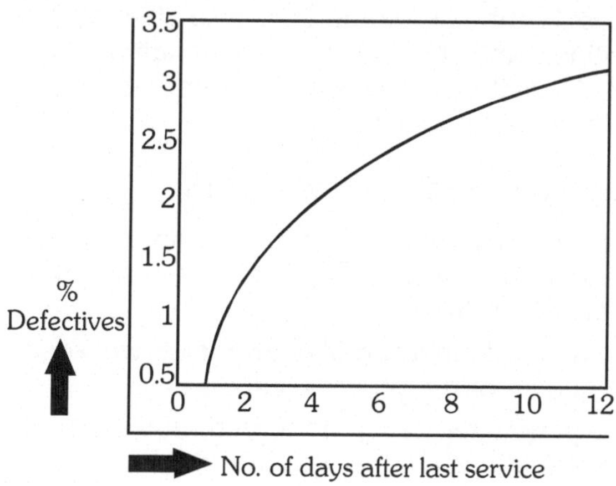

Figure 6.3 Scatter diagram.

The inference may be that this machine must be serviced once a week.

These tools can be used for any type of industry. All employees are nowadays trained in using these tools. Once they have learnt to use these tools, over a period of time, the usefulness of the tools will be reflected in the company's productivity.

6.2.6 Acceptance Sampling

Acceptance sampling is the process of evaluating a small sample of the product in a given lot for the purpose of accepting or rejecting the lot, based on the conformance or non-conformance of the sample to quality specifications. It has a scientific (statistical) basis.

Acceptance quality level (AQL) is the minimum quality level that is considered satisfactory for acceptance. AQL is the maximum percent defective (or number of defective per 100 units) that can be accepted. The probability of acceptance of the lot is high.

6.2.7 Quality Variation and Management Response

There are two kinds of variations that cause a process to drift or deviate from norms :

(a) Random variation (common or inherent variation)

(b) Systemic variation (assignable or special cause variation)

These two kinds of variations call for different managerial responses. Management tries to improve quality by reducing inherent variation. This is done by changing the process itself. The process should not be changed until all assignable variation have been identified and brought under control.

If the process is out – of – control because of an assignable variation, it must be identified and the cause of the variation corrected to bring it under control. Once the process is under control, the process is redesigned to reduce its inherent variability.

6.2.8 Variation is the Enemy of Quality

It seems to be the catchword in many quality management programs. So it seems paradoxical that SQC involves the study of variations. The essence of SQC is to :

- Identify an easily measurable parameter, whose value is important for the quality of the process output.
- Plot the parameter being monitored, in such a way, that the non-random variations can be recognized.
- Decide when to make adjustments to a process.

Control plots, generally known as control charts are used to control variables for attributes like diameter, weight, power- consumption, wetness, etc. The different charts are :

- $\bar{x}$, *R charts* : Direct measurement of process parameters is reflected in these charts.

- *p/np charts* : These charts reflect (Go) / (No – Go) situations. They help in controlling the defectives.
- *C charts* : These charts help in controlling defects.

  Using a control chart, each of the following statistical quality data can be monitored :
  - Single value, mean value
  - Recovery rate
  - Standard deviation
  - Range

Quality assurance is a regulation process. Every analytical series and control sample must undergo the regulation cycle Fig 6.4. at least once :

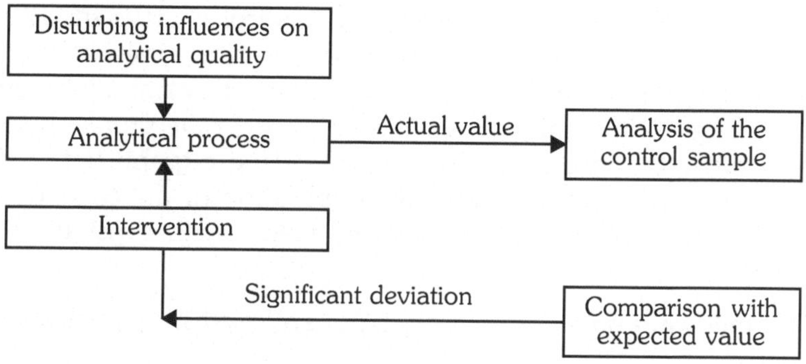

Figure 6.4 Quality regulation cycle.

6.3 The Control Chart System

6.3.1 Principles of a Control Chart

The principle of a control chart is a visual representation of "quality", using as a basis the- desired quantity (expected value of the analysis results for control samples) and the limits

For the latter one distinguishes between warning limits, which if exceeded once still yield tolerable results and control (or action) limits, which if exceeded require immediate action. In a so-called preliminary period, one or more control samples are analyzed in every analysis series.

A precision and — as much as is possible — an accuracy test is then performed on the analytical results for every control sample and compared with established values.

For acceptable analysis quality, the warning and control limits are established and the control charts are constructed.

In the following control period, the adherence to obtained limits is monitored and additional control samples are investigated.

The results of these control analyses, or of the statistical data obtained from them, are continuously entered in the control chart. The abscissa represents the sequence (batch number or working day); results are entered on the ordinate. The progression of results is visible at once; the control chart can be visually evaluated after each additional entry.

The control chart thereby allows the rapid recognition of arising errors, and established control criteria indicate an "out-of-control situation" for the analytical process being monitored.

6.3.2 Types of Control Charts and their Applications

One of the oldest and simplest types of control chart is the Shewhart chart. It be used to monitor the precision of mean values from single results or from multi analyses [2, 3]. Whether or not newly determined value belongs to the entity of values necessary for the preparation of the chart is evaluated visually and objectively using a graph (i.e. results lie within or outside limits or lines) [8]. Application of the chart described here requires a normal distribution and values with constant standard deviation.

The following types of control charts are used in analytical quality assurance :

(i) Shewhart (or conventional) charts as
(ii) x-charts (and blank value charts)
(iii) Recovery rate control charts (RR charts)
(iv) Range control (R-charts)
(v) $\bar{x}$-R combination charts
(vi) Difference charts
(vii) Standard deviation charts
(viii) Cusum charts

Each of these control charts will be described individually below.

6.4 Shewhart Quality Control Chart

The quality control chart, developed by Shewhart (1), is used for industrial product control. The problem consists of a product, which should possess constant features within certain stated limits. The length of a screw represents an example of such a feature. During the manufacturing process, any desired number of items can be spot-checked, i.e. the screws can be measured. When monitoring a characteristic, Shewhart took several random samples within a manufacturing step (e.g. day or machine-dependent period). These n samples then belonged to a subgroup. To prepare the control chart (expected value and establishment of warning and control limits), he then performed analyses on N subgroups Table 6.2. The property in question was also investigated routinely n-times and the corresponding mean was entered into the control chart (Fig. 6.5).

Table 6.2 Table of original values for product control according to Shewhart and related control charts

Measurement number j within the group	**Production step I (= group)**							
	i = 1	2	3	4	.	.	.	N
J = 1	$X_{1,1}$	$X_{2,1}$	$X_{3,1}$		$X_{4,1}$			$X_{N,1}$
J = 2	$X_{1,2}$	.						
J = 3	$X_{1,3}$		.					
J = 4	$X_{1,4}$							
.	.				X			
.						.		
.	.							.
J = n	$X_{1,n}$	.	.	.	.	.		$X_{N,n}$
Group mean	X_1	X_2	.					X_N

Serious changes, which suddenly appear in the production conditions and a slow but steady decline in quality, can be read directly from the graph. Immediate correctional intervention in the production process decreases the risk of “scrap production” and customer complaints.

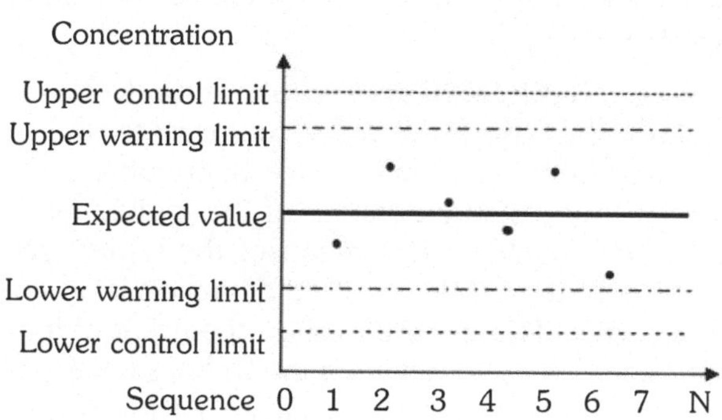

Figure 6.5 Shewart control chart.

Shewhart monitored the measurements not single values of a property, but instead means. This procedure could overwhelm all routine analysis in an analytical laboratory, since control samples must be tested repeatedly for every parameter in every series. Therefore, most of the subgroups described here consist of only one analysis result, i.e. n = 1.

Another fundamental difference to product control in industry is the necessity to produce one's own "control product" (namely control analyses). The actual "product" of an analytical result eludes a precision or accuracy check; at best only a plausibility test can be performed. In addition, the analysis result as "product" may, in an individual case, assume every value within the range. Equivalence with previous or successive results would be pure coincidence for various analysis samples.

6.4.1 Statistical Fundamentals of the Shewhart Chart

If the range obtained by repeated measurements of a sample is divided into classes of uniform size and the frequency with which the individual results fall into a class is counted, then a histogram can be plotted (Fig. 6.6.)

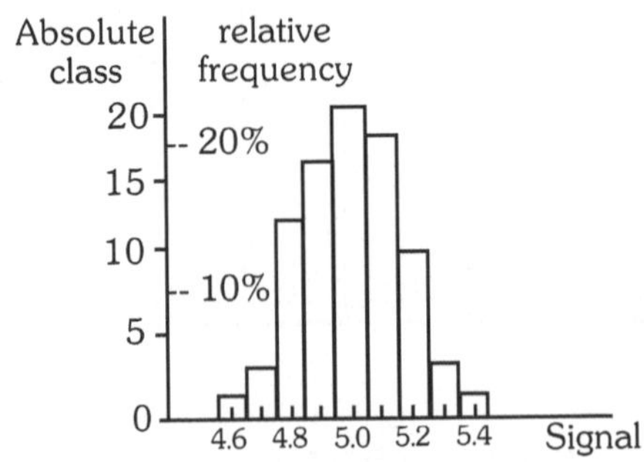

Figure 6.6 Histogram (for small N) (9).

The number of classes is related to the number of individual results (N) : number of classes = vn.

For very frequent repetition of the measurement (N → ∞) and simultaneous; Infinite reduction of the individual classes, the histogram approaches the form of a) called Gaussian (or bell) curve. This normal distribution is described by (the mean value of the individual results, as well as by the standard deviation. The mean of the measurements lies under the peak of the bell curve. The standard deviation is obtained from the intersection of a vertical line drawn through the point of inflection of the curve with the x-axis. The area between the 2s lines covers 68.3 % of the entire area underneath the bell curve and therefore includes 68.3 % of all individual results: the area between the 2s lines covers 95.5 % of the total and the area between the 3s lines 99.7%. Fig. 6.7.

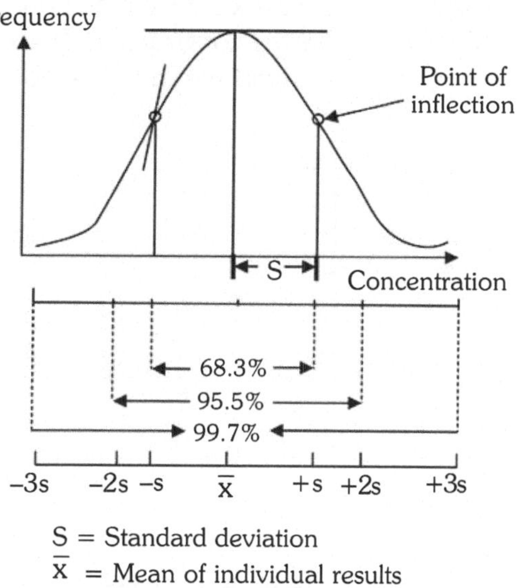

Figure 6.7 Frequency distribution of the analysis results at N $\rightarrow \infty$ repeated analyses and class width $\rightarrow$ 0 (Guassian bell curve).

The following conclusions can be drawn from this representative form:

- The entire area is always the same (= 100%), independent of and s, and ends only in infinity.
- If the results are widely distributed around the mean, i.e. for very large standard deviation, then for the same total area this is represented by a wide but low bell curve.
- Conversely, a narrow, tall curve represents a small standard deviation, i.e. a high degree of precision.

6.4.2 Construction of a Shewhart Chart

The application of control charts in quality assurance is based on the assumption that the obtained results are normally distributed [4]. Shewhart [1] developed therefore a control chart, which features a bell curve turned 90° on its side.

First a system of coordinates is set up in which the ordinate (y-axis) contains the unit of the results and is divided correspondingly (e.g. concentration units). The abscissa (x-axis) is a discreet sequence axis on which the time, series number, day, etc. is recorded in chronological form.

The results of the preliminary period are then entered consecutively.

After N days or series, the mean x and the standard deviation s are calculated and the Shewhart chart is constructed. The central line of the chart is represented by the calculated mean value from the preliminary period (Fig. 6.8).

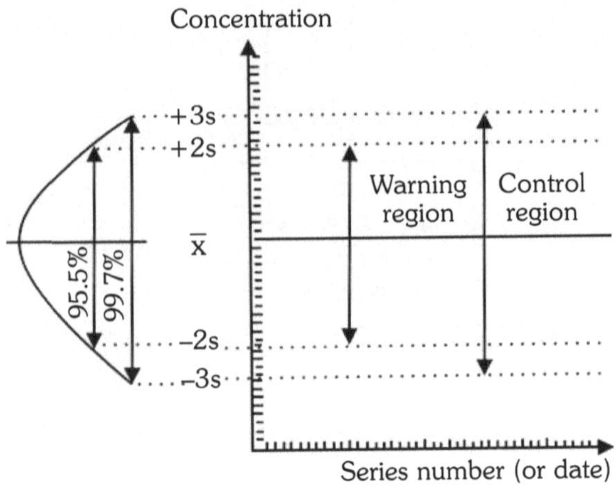

Figure 6.8 Construction or a control chart.

Using the standard deviation, the warning and control limits for $\bar{x} \pm 2s$ resp. $\bar{x} \pm 3s$ are plotted.

Construction aid: the y-axis should always approximately cover the range $\pm$ 4s. That way it is certain that space is available to plot values, which are out of control. The results of the preliminary period are then plotted on the prepared chart and the chart is checked according to the control criteria

The control and warning limits are the $\pm$ 3s and $\pm$ 2s ranges, respectively :

upper control limit UCL = $\bar{x} + 3s$

lower control limit LCL = $\bar{x} - 3s$

upper warning limit UWL = $\bar{x} + 2s$

lower warning limit LWL = $\bar{x} - 2s$

The distance from the +2s line to the –2s line covers 95.5% of the area underneath the curve, i.e. the probability of a "false alarm" in this area is 4.5%, and a single exceeding of these limits is tolerated. The probability of a value exceeding the 3s limit is 0.3 %, i. e. if this occurs, then it is with fair certainty an out of control situation.

During the evaluation of data from the preliminary period, the detection of an out of control situation already present in the preliminary period indicates that corrective measures are urgently required even before beginning the routine analysis.

6.4.3 Evaluation of a Control Chart

The more precise the analytical process is, the more sensitively a control chart reacts, i.e. recognizes out of control situations.

Average Run Length (ARL) and evaluation of control charts

The establishment of limits for control charts occurs with regard to two aspects :

1. Notification of a so-called statistically "out-of-control" situation as rapidly as possible, if the analytical process changes significantly (the measured values belong to another entity!) due to unknown influences on the analytical process (or product, in industrial applications).
2. A small likelihood for a "false alarm", i.e. a measured value which actually belongs to the same entity (the chart), but lies outside the limits incidentally. When the limits chosen are too narrow, one must accept the possibility of false alarms.

An important parameter for the evaluation of control charts and out-of-control situations is the average run length (ARL).

The ARL is defined as the average number of entries on a control chart before a single out-of-control situation appears. [5]

A high ARL (L_0) is necessary if the analytical process is to be in control. The possibility of a "false alarm" (error) is then very small. According to Woodward [5], Lo should be several hundred. For the $\overline{x}$ chart (mean value or conventional control chart), approximately 1 value out of 400 falls outside the 3s limit, even though the procedure is in control- The ARL of the $\overline{x}$ chart is therefore $L_0 = 400$. [6]

On the other hand, an actual out-of-control situation should be indicated as quickly as possible, i.e. the ARL (L_1) must be very small. Goldsmith and Woodward [5] consider a (L_1) between 3 and 10 as reasonable and obtainable with $\overline{x}$ charts.

6.4.4 "Out of Control" Situations

In addition to the detection of large random errors (gross errors), the control chart should also provide hints about systematic errors or trends in systematic errors. The following criteria for out of control situations are normally encountered :

1. One value outside of the control limits.
2. Seven consecutive values on one side of the central line.
3. Seven consecutive values with increasing tendency.
4. Seven consecutive values with decreasing tendency.
5. Two of three consecutive values outside the warning limits.
6. Ten of eleven consecutive values on one side of the central line.

Out of control situations 1 to 4 are depicted in Fig. 6.9.

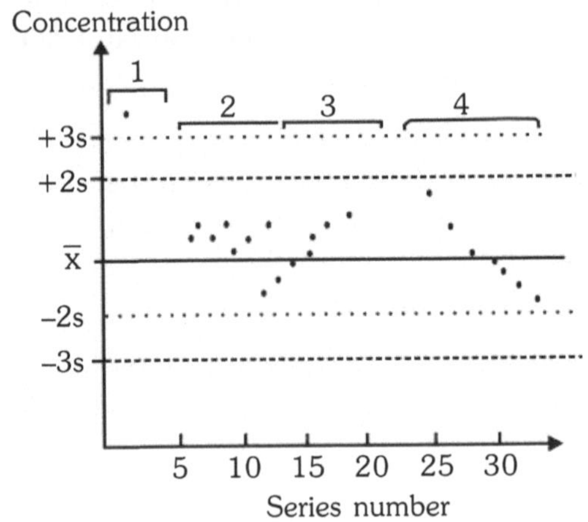

Figure 6.9 Examples of out of control situation.

6.4.5 Conspicuous Entries

When evaluating a control chart, one should not only look for out of control situations but should also follow the general progression of the entries on the chart Figure 6.10 depicts four examples in which at no time is the process "out of control but the order of entries suggest influences that are not random.

Action should be taken even before the appearance of an out of control situations since cases (b), (c) and (d) will lead to "out of control" situations in the nearest future.

(a) Critical changes (cause : rotation of technician, Monday" effect, etc.) (7)

(b) Shift of the mean (cause: technical intervention on the measurement equipment, new reagents, new equipment, disposable articles, etc.)

(c) Trend (cause : equipment influences, aging of reagents, etc.) (7)

(d) Many entries close to the control limits (*s* enlarged).

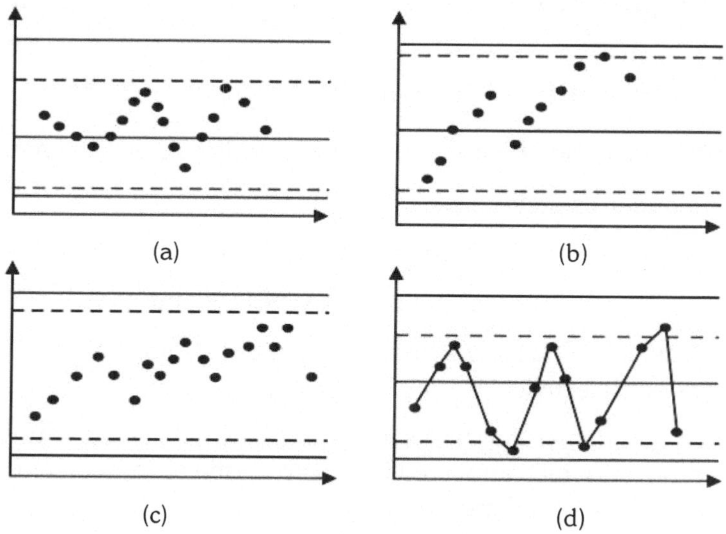

Figure 6.10 Conspicuous order of entries in a Shewhart chart.

6.4.6 Applications of the Shewhart Chart

The Shewhart chart is applied to analytical quality assurance in three different forms :

- $\bar{x}$ - charts
- Blank value charts
- Recovery rate charts

6.5 $\bar{x}$ - charts

The $\bar{x}$ - chart corresponds with the original form of the Shewhart chart for industrial product quality control, except that single values from analytical chemistry are used.

The $\bar{x}$ - chart serves mainly to validation the precision of the process Since systematic changes such as trends can also be detected, the accuracy may also be monitored to a limited extent.

Calibration parameters such as slope and intercept, in so far as they arc determined daily, can also be tested by means of the y-chart. Thus it is possible to use one abscissa (x-axis) for all parameters and to arrange the two ordinates above one another on one page [8].

The choice of control samples is dependent on the quality assurance situation in question and has no influence on the construction of a control chart.

Control samples for an $\overline{x}$ - chart

The following may be used as control samples for an $\overline{x}$ - chart

Pure standard solution

Advantage : Easy to prepare in any desired concentration.

Suitable for validation of the previous calibration.

Disadvantages : Not representative for routine samples. Matrix effects cannot be detected.

If even an original standard sample from the calibration is used, then systematic errors which appeared previously in the calibration also cannot be detected (lack of independence).

Synthetic samples

Advantage : Can be produced by the analyst as needed.

Disadvantages : Preparation is very complicated for more complex matrices since the sample matrix must be simulated. The sample must be stable over time.

Reference samples (Stable natural samples which have been examined thoroughly using other analytical procedures; for example from interlaboratory, or round robin, tests.)

Advantage : More economical than a certified reference material, but also independent.

Disadvantage : Matrix and analyte content may not be representative.

Certified reference material

Advantage : An independent sample with a known expected value. Disadvantages: Relatively expensive and covers only a certain sample matrix, if at all. The analyte content is also not necessarily representative. May be used, however, for monitoring measurement instruments.

A typical data for $\overline{x}$ – chart using standard solution analysis are given in Table 6.3 while the corresponding $\overline{x}$ – charts and Normalized charts are presented in Fig. 6.11 (a) & (b).

Table 6.3 $\overline{x}$ - chart for standard solution

Series number	Results [mg/l]	Deviation [mg/l]	Normalized deviation
1	179.3	–1.00	–0.56
2	179.9	–0.40	–0.22
3	182.6	2.30	1.28
4	180.4	0.10	0.06
5	180.8	0.50	0.28
6	180.9	0.60	0.33
7	179.8	–0.50	–0.28
8	183.7	3.40	1.89
9	178.2	–2.10	–1.17
10	180.9	0.60	0.33
11	178.9	–1.40	–0.78
12	184.5	4.20	2.33
13	181.6	1.30	0.72
14	180.8	0.50	0.28
15	179.0	–1.30	–0.72
16	179.5	–0.80	–0.44
17	178.3	–2.00	1.11
18	177.7	–2.60	–1.44
19	179.3	–1.00	–0.56
20	179.1	–1.20	–0.67
21	182.1	1.80	1.00
22	182.9	2.60	1.44
23	180.3	0.00	0.00
24	178.4	–1.90	–1.06
25	179.0	–1.30	–0.72

Sum : 4507.9
Mean : 180.3
Standard deviation 1.8

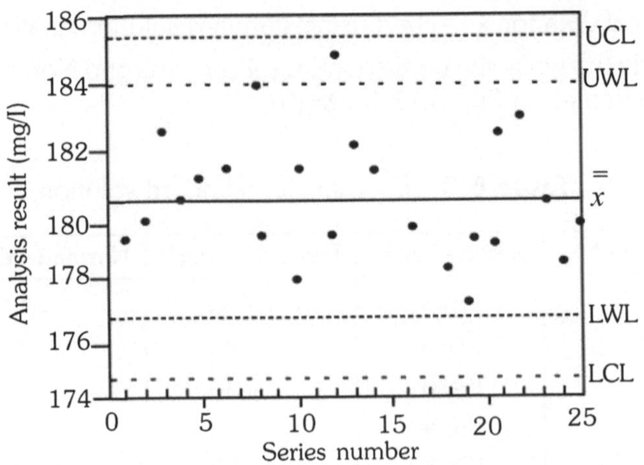

Figure 6.11 (a) RR control chart for a standard of concentration 180 mg/l.

Alternatively, the analytical results may also be entered into a normalized diagram. For this, the deviations of the individual values were calculated and divided by the standard deviation :

$$\text{Normslized deviation} = \frac{\text{Individual value} - \text{Mean}}{\text{Standard deviation}}$$

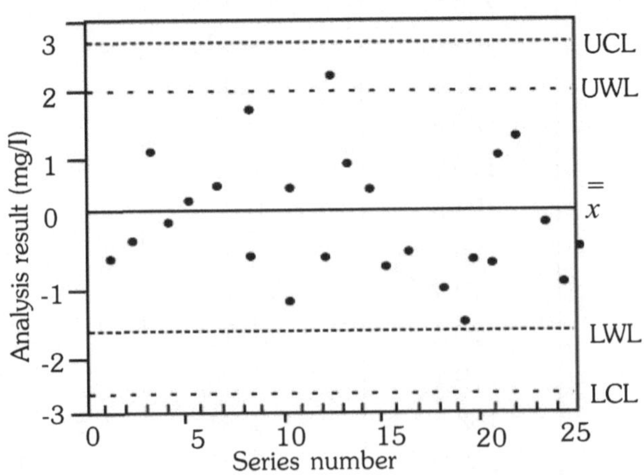

Figure 6.11 (b) Normalized $\overline{x}$ -chart.

6.6 Blank Value Charts

The blank value chart (Fig. 6.12) is a special application of the $\overline{x}$ - chart. It provides special information on the reagent and measurement systems used.

Special feature : Measured values and not results (i.e. concentrations) are entered into the blank value chart.

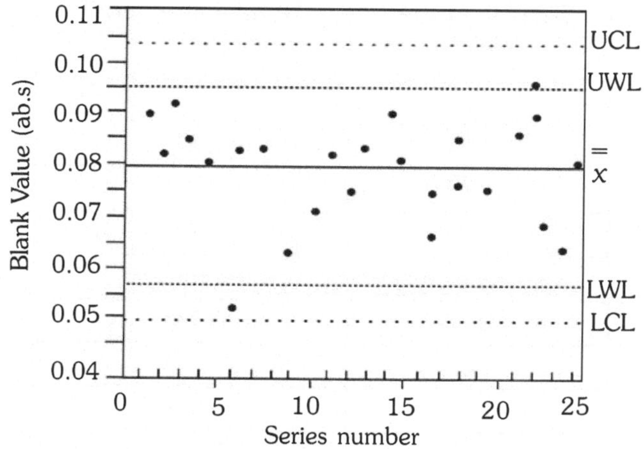

Figure 6.12 Blank value control chart.

6.6.1 Scope of the Blank Control

Information about the scope of the blank analyses to be performed must be made before establishing the decision criteria.(Table 6.4).

Table 6.4

Series number	Blank value [abs]
1	0.089
2	0.080
3	0.091
4	0.083
5	0.079
6	0.054
7	0.081
8	0.082
9	0.065
10	0.073
11	0.080
12	0.073
13	0.081
14	0.089

Table 6.4 *Contd...*

Series number	Blank value [abs]
15	0.079
16	0.076
17	0.069
18	0.083
19	0.076
20	0.075
21	0.083
22	0.097
23	0.068
24	0.066
25	0.079

In order to be correct, the simultaneous determination of the blank value would be required for each analysis; this requirement cannot be met because it is very labor and cost intensive, it appears sensible to determine a minimum of two blank values per analysis series, whereby one is determined at the beginning and the second at the end of the series. Such an arrangement has, in addition to the precise determination of the blank value, the advantage that a drift check can also be performed. The arithmetic mean of n individual blank values per analysis series can be used to maintain the blank value chart. The limits are determined according to using the standard deviation of the mean.

$$S_{\bar{x}} = \frac{S}{\sqrt{n}}$$

6.6.2 Maintaining a Blank Value Chart

The control and warning limits are determined by means of the -C'-chart from the results of the analyses done in the preliminary period.

All further decision criteria, i. e. proof of high or low mean blank values and detection of trends, are the same as those for $\bar{x}$ - charts.

6.7 Recovery Rate Control Charts

General Analyses of control samples and the management of $\bar{x}$ - charts provide no information about errors caused by matrix influences in the sample. Errors caused by the inclusion of other substances contained in the sample matrix should be especially rare for analyses, which put particular emphasis on the specificity of the process (and therefore on the accuracy of the results).

The analytical process may be tested for matrix influences by determining the recovery rate (RR) of spiked actual samples.

The results on the standard sample can also be used for a RR control chart : Fig. 6.13.

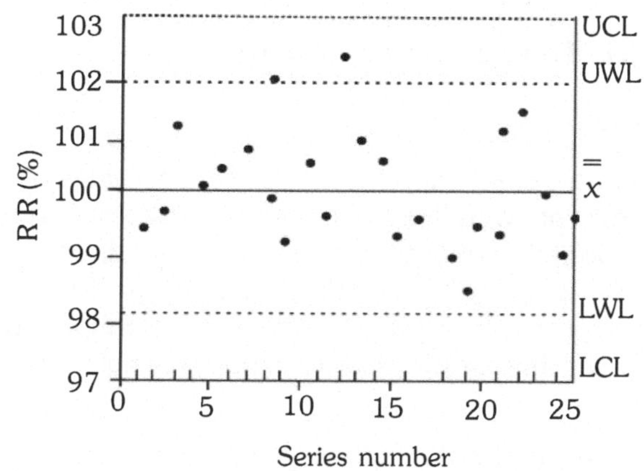

Figure 6.13 RR control chart for a standard of concentration 180 mg/l.

$$RR = \frac{\text{Results}}{180 \text{ mg/l}} \times 100\%$$

The central line was defined as a 100% recovery rate.

However, the recovery rate detects only matrix-dependent proportional systematic errors; constant systematic errors remain undetected when spiking. In this case the recovery rate is calculated as follows :

$$\left(RR = \frac{\text{Actual increase of analysis value}}{\text{Expected increase}}\right).100\%$$

$$\left(= \frac{x_{\text{spiked}} - x_{\text{unspiked}}}{\Delta x_{\text{expected}}}\right) \times 100\%$$

Therefore the determination of the recovery rate is limited as a control of accuracy. In exceptional cases trueness may be checked by calculating the recovery rate, but then only if synthetic samples or reference samples or certified reference materials having known expected values (x_{exp}) are used.

The analysis of such certified reference materials produces an analysis value x_{actual}.

The recovery rate can then be calculated as follows :

$$RR = \left(\frac{x_{act}}{x_{exp}}\right) . 100\%$$

The quality target should have a recovery rate of approximately 100%, since only there are systematic matrixes influenced are completely asserted.

6.8 R-chart (Range Control Chart)

6.8.1 General

While the Shewhart chart shows how well mean values of subgroups or single values correlate with the grand average (process mean), it does not provide any information about the distribution of individual results within and between the subgroups. In contrast, the R-chart (.R = range) serves above all the purpose of precision control. For this range is defined as the difference between the largest and the smallest single result for multiple analyses.

The R-chart is used for the following control possibilities :

1. ***Precision control***

   A fundamental requirement for the use of Shewhart charts is the constancy of the standard deviations. The R-chart can detect significant differences between the standard deviation of the subgroups [4] and represents therefore a test of the variance homogeneity.

2. ***Limited accuracy control - drift control***

   Trends within a series and equipment drifts may be monitored by means of an R-chart, which has been modified to a difference chart.

   Charts are only useful if the control limits are not set by outside factors, but result from the imprecision of the analysis.

6.8.2 Establishment of an R-chart

In order to establish an R-chart, the following quantities must be known or calculated :

- number n of repeated measurements per subgroup (n_2), at least n = 2.
- number N of subgroups.

- R_i range of subgroup i.
- $\overline{R}$, mean value of ranges.
- (s^2, variance of the entire measurement).
- upper warning limit UWL.
- lower warning limit LWL.
- upper control limit UCL.
- lower control limit LCL.

The ranges R_i, of all subgroups must be determined and then combined as $\overline{R}$:

R_i = largest value - smallest value of a subgroup i consisting of n single measurements

$$\overline{R} = \frac{\Sigma R_i}{N}$$

$\overline{R}$ forms the "central line" of the -R-chart (Fig. 6.14.)

The respective warning and control limits are obtained from the mean range R by multiplying it with a factor D, which is a function of the number of multiple determinations n and the significance level :

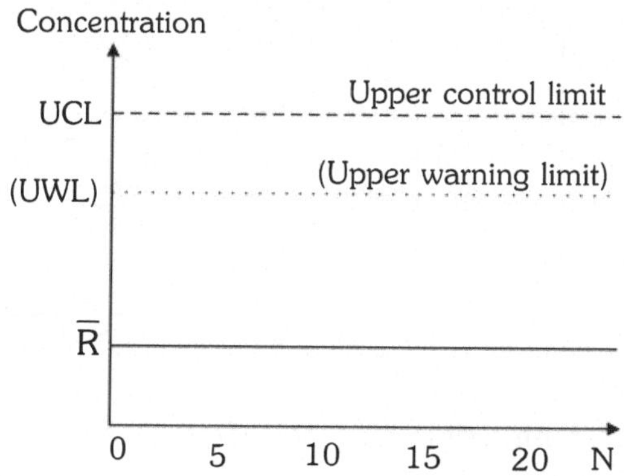

Figure 6.14 R – chart (range chart) with lower limits at zero.

6.8.3 Out of Control Situations

The decision criteria described for Shewhart charts can only conditionally serve as decision criteria for R-charts.

For example, it is not reasonable to assume an out of control situation if seven consecutive values lie underneath the center line $\overline{R}$. This could possibly imply just the opposite - an improvement of the precision. If such a situation were to continue, then it is recommended that the control limits be recalculated.

Decision criteria for R-charts :

An out of control situation exists if,

- R_i lies above the upper control limit (Fig. 6.15.).
- R_i, lies below the lower control limit (valid only if LCL > 0).
- seven consecutive values show an increasing «r decreasing tendency.
- seven consecutive values lie above the range mean R (Fig. 6.15).

Similarly, if at least one R, in the preliminary period lies outside the upper control limit, all quantities required for the establishment of an R-chart must be recalculated. Cyclical movements [increasing (Fig. 6.15.) or decreasing] of the ranges indicate influences resulting from the maintenance schedule of the instruments ageing of the reagent [7]. However, this is not an out of control situation.

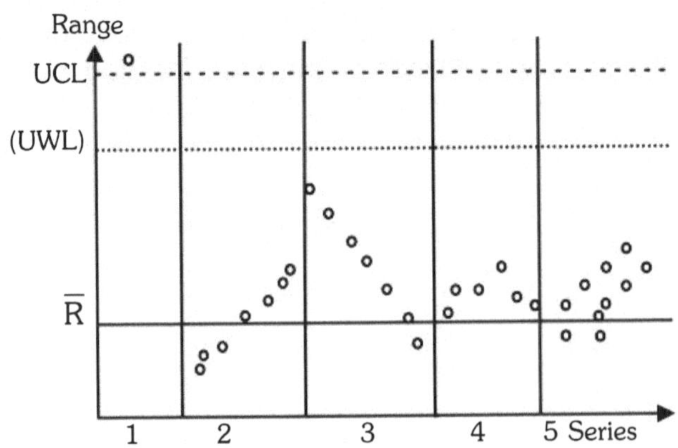

Figure 6.15 Out-of-control situations for R-charts.

6.8.4 Applications of R-charts

For practical applications in analytical laboratories the R-chart appears only in its simplest form, i.e. only one duplicate determination per analysis series. A larger number of parallel determinations would indeed result in a more sensitive precision control, however the effort required for n > 2 is usually not acceptable.

6.8.5 Control Samples for R-charts

Establishing R-charts by means of standard samples or control samples with known content is of little value since the - chart can provide sufficient information instead.

Analysis of standard reference materials also has definite disadvantages, which do not occur with actual samples. Matrix influences, deviations in the stability of the sample, etc. are only registered in quality assurance through the use of actual samples. The precision is therefore verified under conditions close to reality.

Whitby [9] logically recommends that duplicate determinations be performed on actual samples as often as possible. At the beginning of each analysis series one of the actual samples is declared a "control sample" and it is analyzed again at the end of the series (in all, a duplicate determination).

It must be taken into account that the actual samples lie within a concentration range, since the standard deviation and also the ranges are often concentration dependent [9, 10] (Table 6.5). Should an R-chart be maintained independently of the concentration, then the perceptual relative range must be related to it [10]. At the least, changing the measuring or display range will result in a significant change of precision.

Table 6.5 Concentration dependent ranges

X_{i1}	X_{i2}	R_i	x_i	$R_i / x_i \cdot 100\%$
11.2	11.10	0.2	11.1	1.80%
23.5	24.0	0.5	23.75	2.11%
114.3	112.0	2.3	113.15	1.24%
69.3	70.7	1.4	70.0	2.00 %
78.7	80.3	1.6	79.5	2.01 %
100.5	102.5	2.0	101.5	1.97%
203.4	198.8	4.6	201.1	2.29%
54.7	55.8	1.1	55.25	1.99%
150.1	153.1	3.0	151.6	1.98%
90.8	89.0	1.8	89.9	2.00%

$R = 1.85$

$x = 89.685$

6.8.6 Example for Concentration Dependent Ranges

The R-values listed in Table 6.5 have been represented graphically using the means (Fig. 6.16). The R, values are obviously dependent on the concentration. The correlation coefficient amounts to,

$$r = \frac{\Sigma\left(\bar{x}_i - \bar{\bar{x}}\right).\left(R_i - \bar{R}\right)}{\sqrt{\Sigma\left(\bar{x}_i - \bar{\bar{x}}\right)^2 .\left(R_i - \bar{R}\right)^2}} = 09941$$

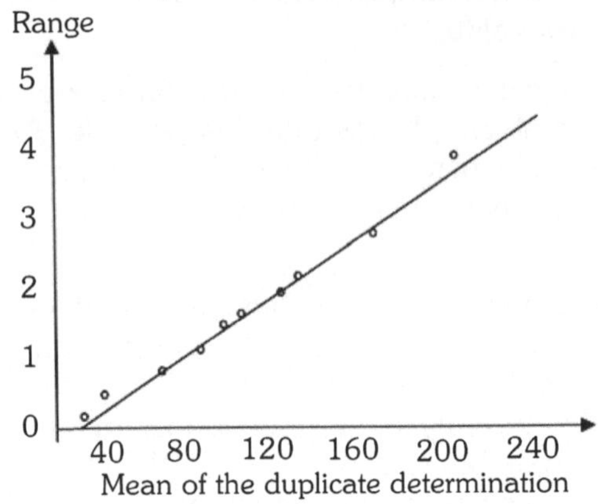

Figure 6.16 Dependence of the ranges on concentration, mean value of the duplicate determination.

Dependence between the range (y-values) and the concentration (x-values) can be proven statistically if the correlation coefficient r is significantly different from zero. To test this, the value of r at f = n — 2 degrees of freedom is compared with the threshold value r (P = 99 %, *f*). If ½ r ½ > r (P = 99 %, *f*), then a dependence exists. In the example r = 0.9941 is larger than r (P = 99%, *f* = 8) = 0.77 which certifies that the range is dependent on concentration.

6.9 $\bar{x}$– R combination Charts

The $\bar{x}$-R combination chart is probably the most useful control chart used in industrial quality assurance [4]. It consists of an $\bar{x}$-chart and an R-chart together arranged so that mean value and range for one given subgroup are positioned above one another on the graph (Fig. 6.17).

This process allows different changes to be recorded simultaneously on one chart. The $\bar{x}$-chart reacts sensitively to changes in the mean value of the subgroups; in contrast the R-chart provides information about too large a distribution within the subgroup.

The primary advantage of this method is that it enables one to decide whether the deviation between subgroups is significantly larger than [the deviation within a subgroup. In this situation, the R-chart is in control and the $\overline{x}$ - chart indicates "out of control" situations [9], This occurs frequently with certain chemical processes indicating insufficiently controlled variables (e.g. temperature).

If the opposite situation occurs, i.e. the-r-chart is in control and the R-chart is out of control, or if a trend is spoiled, this indicates a change in the individual variances [7].

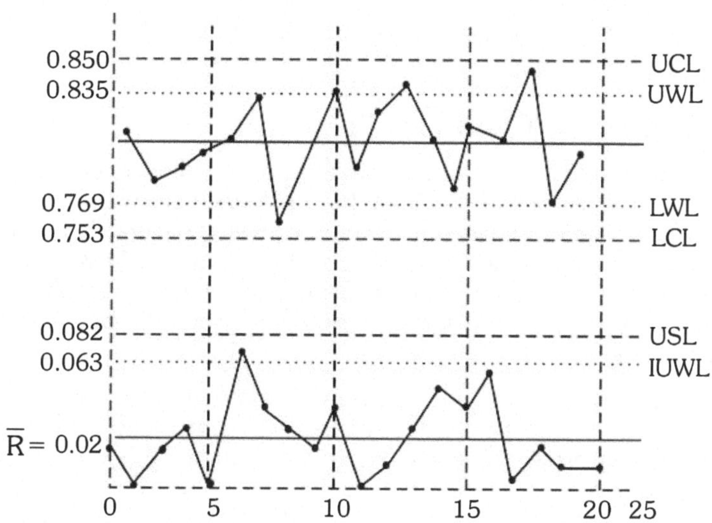

Figure 6.17 $\overline{x}$ - R combination chart.

If the mean values tend to always move in the same direction as the range, it could be a "skewed" distribution (7) (the same is true for continuous movement in the opposite direction).

The $\overline{x}$ -R chart only makes sense if the same control sample is used for both range and mean value control. A control sample (synthetic or natural), which remains stable over a long period of time, is required.

The maintaining of a matrix-representative $\overline{x}$ -R chart is especially recommended for the regular analysis of multiple similar samples within an analysis series. The minimum required duplicate determination of a control sample per matrix increases the total analysis effort significantly and is not justifiable if only a few of the samples within the series have the same matrix (Fig. 6.18). For example, the additional control analysis effort required decreases to < 10% only for a series of 20 or more samples.

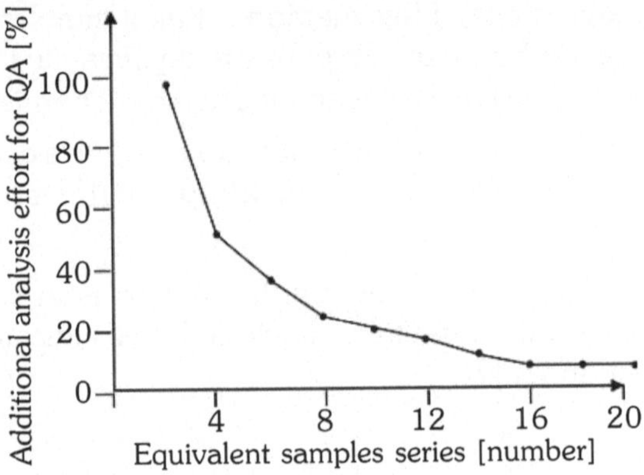

Figure 6.18 Additional analysis effort for the $\overline{x}$ - R chart.

6.10 Difference Chart [11, 9]

While the R-chart uses the absolute value of the difference between the largest and smallest analysis values, the difference chart uses the amount of the difference including its sign. The objective is specifically the detection of systematic errors, which first appear during an analysis series. For a difference chart, an actual sample from each series is analyzed twice. As many analyses from the series as possible should lie between the two determinations.

The differences $d_i = x_{i2} - x_{i1}$, whereby the first value must always be subtracted from the second value, are entered onto a control chart while observing the appropriate signs. The central line of this chart represents the expected value of the differences, i.e. the value zero. Under optimal conditions, the differences must be distributed around the zero-line according to their signs. If a drift is present (for example from the equipment), x_2 will become ever larger (or smaller) than x_i, which is documented by a lop-sided position of the differences above (or below) the zero line (Fig. 6.19).

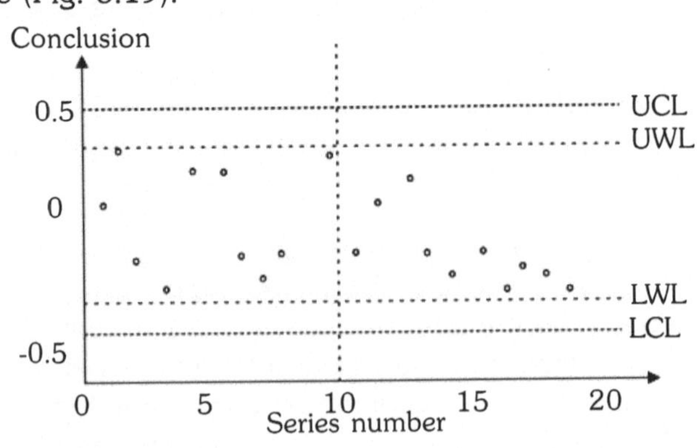

Figure 6.19 Difference chart showing the presence of drift calculation of control limits.

The control limits are calculated

(a) From the standard deviation s_d [11]

$$S_d = \sqrt{\frac{\Sigma d_i^{\,2} - \frac{(\Sigma d_i^{\,2})^2}{N}}{N-1}}$$

Mean = 0, Warning limit : $\pm$ 2 S_d, Control limit : $\pm$ 3S_d

Since s_d is dependent on the concentration, this control chart may only be used for samples which lie within a limited concentration range!

(b) Using the mean range $\bar{R}$

$$\bar{R} = \frac{\Sigma R_1}{N}$$

Mean = 0, Warning limit : 1.77.R (compare with 2s), Control limit: 2.65. R (compare with 3s).

6.10.1 Control Samples for the Difference Chart

An absolute requirement for maintaining a difference chart is the use of stable control samples. Their choice is determined by the monitoring objective.

If only the measuring instrument (detection step) is to be monitored, then unknown matrix errors must be ruled out. Only standards which undergo the actual measurement may be considered as control samples. This procedure is comparable to measurements for instrument adjustment.

Stable actual samples are required to monitor the entire analytical process. As an alternative to synthetic samples and stable natural samples, which serve as control samples over a longer period of time, ;m actual sample from the analysis series HI question may be used (similarly 10 range control). However, it must be certain that the sample undergoes no physical, chemical or biological changes during the lime period between the two control analyses.

6.11 Standard Deviation Chart (s-chart)

This chart is used in a way similar to the R-chart to monitor the distribution of the basic entity. The s-chart, however, is better suited for subgroup sizes of n > 10 than is the R-chart. Used in combination with a mean value chart, the r-chart is able to detect systematic errors quickly [12].

Calculation of the central line and control limits for the s-chart

The central line is entered as the mean standard deviation (s_w)

$$S_w = \sqrt{\frac{\sum_{i=1}^{N} f_i \cdot s_i^2}{\sum_{i=1}^{N} f_i}} = \sqrt{\frac{\sum_{i=1}^{N} (n_i - 1) \cdot s_i^2}{\sum_{i=1}^{N} (n_i - 1)}}$$

or for duplicate determinations ($n_i = 2$) :

$$S_w = \sqrt{\frac{\Sigma S_i^2}{N}}$$

The control limits are obtained from the x^2 distribution using table values x^2 (n – 1; α / 2) and x^2 (n – 1; 1 – α / 2).

$$LCL = s_w \cdot \sqrt{1/n-1. X^2 \; (n-1;\alpha/2)}$$

$$UCL = s_w \cdot \sqrt{1/n-1. X^2 \; (n-1;1-\alpha/2)}$$

Table 6.6 Threshold values of the x^2 distribution for α = 1 %

n – 1	**α / 2 = 0.5%**	**1 – α / 2 = 99.5 %**
1 *	$3.93 \,.\, 10^{-5}$	7.879
2	$1.00 .\, 10^{-2}$	10.60
3	$7.17 \text{-} 10^{-2}$	12.84
4	0.207	14.86
5	0.412	16.75

*Corresponds to a duplicate determination (n = 2)

6.12 Cusum Chart

6.12.1 Principle of the Cusum Chart

The cumulative sum S (cusum) is understood [o be the sum of the errors from one target value [13]. The target value may, for example, be the mean value of a control sample determined in the preliminary period. This mean value, also known as the reference value is subtracted from every control analysis x_i, and the difference is added to the sum of all previous differences [14].

Cumulative sums :

$$S_1 = (x_1 - k)$$
$$S_2 = S_1 + (x_2 - k)$$
$$S_3 = S_2 + (x_3 - k)$$
$$SN = S_{N-1} + (x_n - k) = (\Sigma\, x_c - nk)$$

The cusum value S_N (ordinate) is then plotted against the number of observed results N (abscissa) on a control chart.

To determine an out of control situation, the slope of the cusum line is evaluated (Fig. 6.20). If the process is in control, the results of the control analysis vary randomly around the reference value k, and the cumulative sums are distribute around the value 0. A change in the process leads to an increase or decrease in the cumulative sum, the slope of the cusum line changes, and an out of control situation is detected.

6.12.2 Purpose and Applications of the Cusum Chart

The cusum chart was introduced to industrial quality assurance by E.S. Page [15] in 1954. This chart is a further development of the Shewhart chart, whereby single results are no longer entered but instead the summation of the deviations of the single results from a set value.

Therefore each new entry contains not only information about the current status but also about-past analysis values of the analytical process in question. [2]

In this manner, changes which would not lead to an out of control situation on an $\overline{x}$-chart can be more easily detected. This is especially advantageous for processes with a large variance.

The cusum technique is especially suited to the following applications :

- Recognition of a systematic change or shift in the mean value of a process in progress (15).
- Determination of the order of magnitude by which the mean value has changed [15].
- Determination of the moment the change occurred [15].
- Prediction of the future mean value on short notice [5]

6.12.3 Establishing a Cusum Chart

A cusum chart should be dimensioned so that it reacts sensitively to the smallest deviation in the mean value that is seen as important in practice.

This reaction should be reflected in a clearly visible change in the slope of the cusum line. In the case of an "in control process", the slope of the line is decisively dependant upon the chose reference vale "*k*"; in the case of an "out of control process", the clearness of the change in the slope is dependant on the scale of the Y – axis (cusum axis). Therefore one must keep in mind not only a correct choice of the reference vale *k*, but of the scale factor "*w*" as well.

6.12.4 Choice of the Reference Value "*k*"

If a certified reference material is available for use in quality assurance, then the given standard concentration is equivalent to the reference value k. If this is not the case, the concentration of the control sample must be determined in a preliminary period. Estimation of the mean values should be made based on at least 20 replicates.

If the reference value *k* is imprecisely determined then the cusum values do not deviate around the value "0", i.e the cusum line rises or falls continuously. An example is shown in the Fig. 6.20.

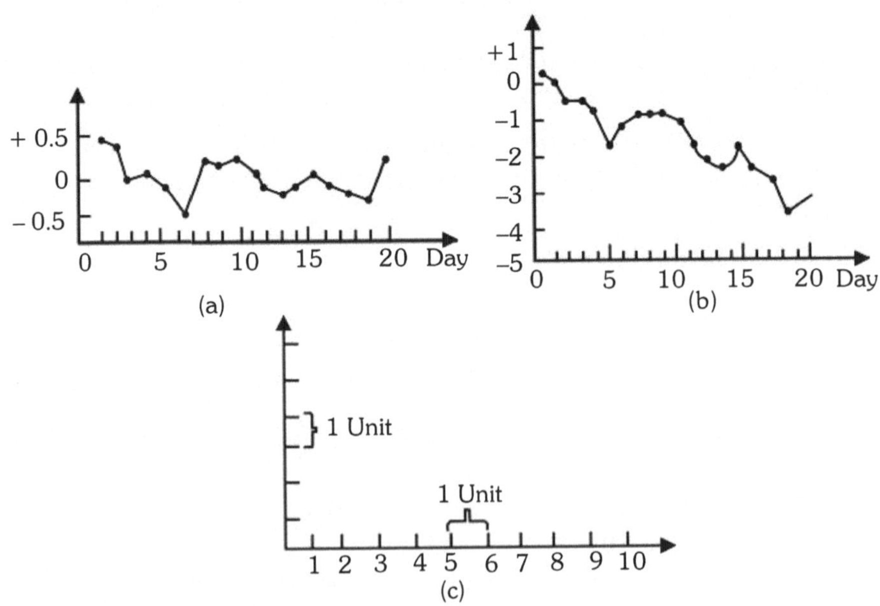

Figure 6.20 Cusum Progression.

(a) Cusum progression for a properly chosen reference value $k = 6.0$.

(b) Cusum progression for an incorrect reference value $k = 6.2$.

(c) Scale of the cusum axis.

If the "correct" reference value is not chosen, then the upper or lower limits of the cusum chart may be reached quite quickly and small changes in slope are more difficult to determine.

6.12.5 Scale of the Y–Axis (Cusum Axis)

At first the abscissa and ordinate are assigned at equidistant divisions (each designated as one unit). The scale of the axes is determined by the scale factor "w" which indicates cusum value corresponds with a unit on the cusum axis. Normally "w" is expressed as "q – number of standard deviations". For this the standard deviation "s" is determined from the preliminary period standard deviation s'. for only one control analysis per series s = s'; if the cusum chart is constructed with mean values from each of n analyses, then the standard deviation of the mean values is included in the scale :

$$s = \frac{s'}{\sqrt{n}}$$

Both the scale of the cusum axis and the correct or skillful) choice of the reference value contributes to a cusum chart which is easier to use. The cusum axis dimensions should neither be too far apart nor too close together; a change in the slope is difficult to determine in both cases (Fig. 6.21).

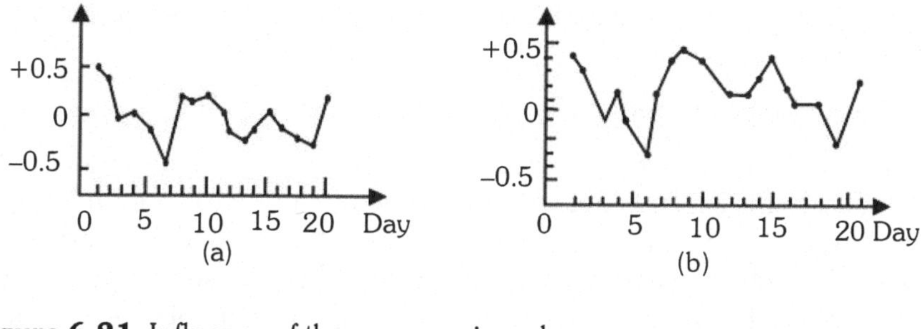

Figure 6.21 Influence of the cusum axis scale.

(a) Suitable choice of scale ($w = 2s$)

(b) Scale increments too far apart.

Goldsmith and Whitfield and Ewan recommended a scale factor of "w" = 2s (q = 2) to w = 1s (q = 1) for use with graphic decision criteria. If the distance between two entries on the axis (e. g. one day)is defined as a unit, then the same distance on the cusum axis is represented by 2s. the cusum line increases by 45° if two consecutive values differentiate by 2s.

6.12.6 Determination of an Out of Control Situation

In order to determine an out of control situation, there are three decision criteria for cusum charts :

Visual decision criterion.

The V – mask as decision criterion.

Numerical decision criterion. (this corresponds to the V – mask standardized conditions)

6.12.6.1 *Visual decision criterion*

A deviation of the actual from the required mean value leads to a change in slope. This change can be easily determined visually if the chart is properly dimensioned and the process is reliable. However, only slight changes in the cusum progression make a visual interpretation difficult. In order to make decisions, which can be reproduced by others, it is advantageous to use an objective decision criterion.

6.12.6.2 *V – mask*

The v – mask, developed by Barnard (17) Barnard G.A., Charts and stochostics Bolum J.R. Statist. Soc. B 21 (1950) 239-27 in 1959 is a two – sided statistical test, which can determine positive and negative deviations from a mean value. Since it is possible to consider the previous cusum progression, the V – mask technique combines visual interpretation with objective test criteria.

The V – mask is defined by the two parameters d & θ.

The leading distance d represents the distance from the vertex of the V – mask to the most recent entry on the chart; d is expressed in abscissa (e. g. days). θ is the angle between the arms of the mask and the horizontal drawn through the mask vertex. After establishing these two parameters, the V – mask may be drawn on transparent film or a cut out of a cardboard.

The V – mask is then positioned on the cusum chart at a distance d from the most recent entry so that the vertex (placed horizontally) points forward. For each new entry, the mask is shifted so that the point E comes to lie on the new cusum value. This represents a shifting of one abscissa unit. It should be noted that the V – mask may not turn its vertex around, i.e., the leading distance d remains parallel to the x – axis. An out of control situation is indicated if the cusum line process – one of the arms of the V – mask. The larger θ and d are, the more infrequent an out of control situation occurs.

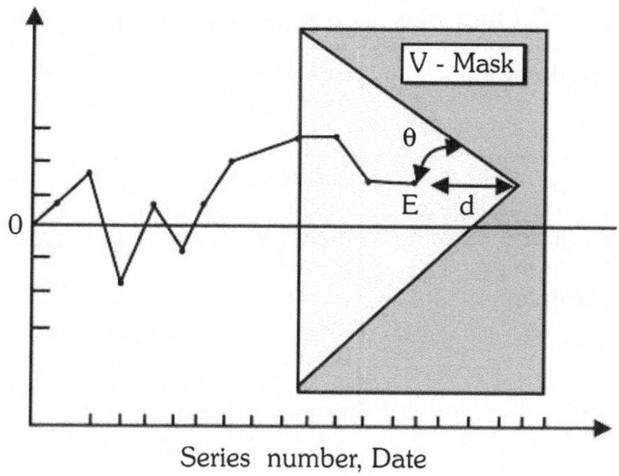

Figure 6.22 V – mask and parameters *d* and θ.

If the cusum line cuts through the upper arm of the mask, then the mean value has decreased. The mean value has increased if the line crosses the lower arm.

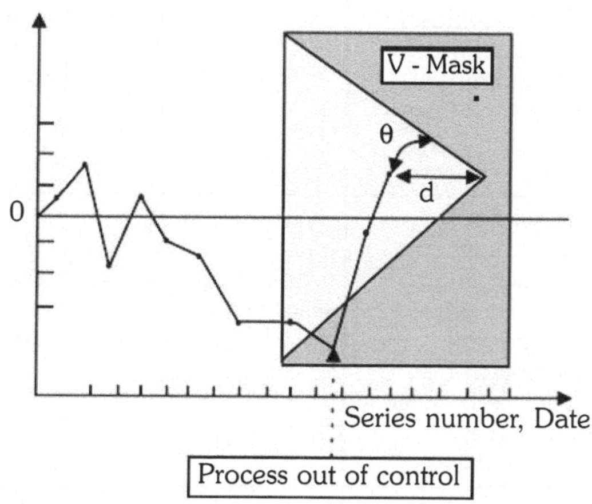

Figure 6.23 Out of control situation.

The first cusum value which lies outside the V – mask indicates the time point at which the out of control situation appeared. This information can be very helpful when searching for the cause of the error. If the error is discovered and corrected, then the cumulative summation begins again at zero.

The Overview of frequently used control charts in quality assurance are given in Table 6.7.

Table 6.7 Overview of frequently used control charts

Type of control chart	Calculations	Suitable for detecting	Required analyses
x-chart	Mean value and standard deviation, control and warning limits in the preliminary	Gross errors (deviation from the mean), systematic errors (trends, changes in the mean), random errors (scatter of individual values), generally for precision control)	Control sample analyses at regular intervals
Difference chart	Mean difference, standard deviation and control limits in the preliminary period; differences obtained from control sample analyses	Instrument drift	At least two determination for each control sample at established intervals at the beginning and end of a series.
R-chart (range chart)	Mean range, standard deviation and control limits in the preliminary period; range from control sample analyses	Imprecision	At least two determination for actual control sample at established intervals
Recovery rate (RR) chart	Mean RR, standard deviation, control warning limits in the preliminary period; calculation of the RR from the results of the control sample analyses	Inaccuracy, proportional systematic errors	At least one analysis of each an unspiked control or actual sample for a known spiking quantity.
Blank control chart	Mean and standard deviation, control warning limits in the preliminary period;	Control of the blank values, errors in measuring instruments, reagent deviations.	At least two blank value determinations at established intervals.
Cusum chart	Reference value and standard deviation from the preliminary period; Setting the leading distance and half angles of the V- mask; calculation of the cumulative sum	Inaccuracy, drift	Control sample analyses at established intervals

Summary

Statistical process control techniques helps in controlling the manufacturing processes more effectively. These techniques monitor the manufacture process and control the quality of these processes. Manufacturers can stop the flow in the production line if and when it is required in case any anomalies are to be corrected or if they find that the process is deviating from norms.

In other words, SQC is a method to improve product quality, thereby limiting waste and rework. Naturally, production also increases.

The term 'statistical' method implies the collection of numerical data, which are tabulated, and summarized using prescribed statistical tools for the purpose of analysis and reporting.

Statistical process control

According to Deming, the American 'Quality Guru', Quality in production can be achieved by:

Identifying the causes of production problems

Carefully monitoring production to stop errors before too many products are made.

Deming divides the causes of problems into two categories – Common and Special causes. Common causes are systemic problems, common to the system and shared by many workers, machines and product types. Special causes are problems that relate to individual workers, machines or material shipments.

Statistical process control tools

SPC can be applied by following a sequence of steps

At each stage, there are statistical tools that can be used. The steps and the corresponding tools are:

Define the problem, identify primary causes, and prioritize areas to receive follow up attention (Pareto chart).

Determine the level of process control and the process capability of the primary possible process by the direct measurements from the operation (Control charts).

Identify potential causes of instability identified in the previous stage. (Fishbone diagram or Cause and effect diagram).

Quantify the relationship between the variables (process or product) of interest from the previous step and other process variables (Scatter diagram, and correlation studies).

Confirm the effect of any process or equipment changes on process stability and capability (Control charts).

We can use Control charts to identify the extent of deviations that occur in the processes. Control charts are line graphs that record the number of defects. A control chart plots sampled data, representing process output, with respect to time, in a form that makes it easy to analyse whether the process is in control or out of control.

Quality variation and Management response

There are two kinds of variations that cause a process to drift or deviate from norms:

Random variation (common or inherent variation)

Systemic variation (assignable or special cause variation)

These two kinds of variations call for different managerial responses. Management tries to improve quality by reducing inherent variation. This is done by changing the process itself. The process should not be changed until all assignable variation have been identified and brought under control.

If the process is out – of – control because of an assignable variation, it must be identified and the cause of the variation corrected to bring it under control. Once the process is under control, the process is redesigned to reduce its inherent variability.

Variation is the enemy of quality It seems to be the catchword in many quality management programs. So it seems paradoxical that SQC involves the study of variations. The essence of SQC is to:

Identify an easily measurable parameter, whose value is important for the quality of the process output. Plot the parameter being monitored, in such a way, that the non-random variations can be recognized.

Decide when to make adjustments to a process.

Control plots, generally known as control charts are used to control variables for attributes like diameter, weight, power-consumption, wetness, etc. The different charts are:

$\bar{x}$ ***, R charts :*** Direct measurement of process parameters is reflected in these charts.

p/np charts : These charts reflect (Go) / (No – Go) situations. They help in controlling the defectives.

C charts : These charts help in controlling defects.

Using a control chart, each of the following statistical quality data can be monitored:

- Single value, mean value
- Recovery rate
- Standard deviation
- Range

Questions

1. What is meant by statistical quality control? Discuss applicable statistical process control tools?
2. What are the statistical process control tools? Explain the various statistical process control tools?
3. What is the control chart system? Explain the principle in detail? Explain various types of quality control charts?
4. How do you construct Shewhart charts?
5. How control charts are equated?
6. What are $\overline{x}$ charts?
7. What are blank value charts? What are its blanks?
8. What are Recovery charts?
9. What are Range control charts?
10. What are $\overline{x}$ – R control charts?
11. What are the different charts and statistical deviations? Discuss its applications?
12. What is a Cusum chart? Describe in detal in its applications?

7

Quality Audit

7.1 What is Quality Audit ?

Quality Audit is defined as "A systematic and independent examination to determine whether quality activities and related results comply with planned arrangements and whether these arrangements are implemented effectively and are suitable to achieve objectives.

It should be noted that the audit checks compliance with planned arrangements and implementation of these arrangements. The decision as to whether these arrangements are suitable to achieve objectives is with the management personnel who receive and review the audit reports. NOT the auditor.

As defined then, an audit is an information gathering activity so that the need for improvement or corrective action may be evaluated. There is no element of a witch hunt or apportioning blame for problems. It is important to establish this fact amongst auditees because defensiveness is not conducive to information flow.

Audits may be internal or external and do not necessarily have to cover the whole system at once but may cover elements of it. Independence is ensured by the auditors having no direct responsibility in the audited area but preferably working in co-operation with the relevant personnel.

The first party audit is an audit carried out by an organisation on itself, i.e. an internal audit. Note that this is not necessarily on one site; internal audits can be carried out on overseas sites, for example.

A second party audit is an audit by one organisation, working on its own behalf, on another. This is usually an audit on a supplier by a customer.

Third party audit is an audit by an Independent organisation (the third party) on a supplier. This may be done at the request of a group of customers.

Although audits, auditing and auditors are synonymous with assessments. It may be considered that an audit is an examination of a single activity, element, department etc., whereas an assessment is a collection of such audits.

7.2 Types of Audit

There are several types of audit :

(a) *Adequacy audit / Document review :*

This is also known as a system or management audit and is normally an office exercise which determines the extent to which the documented system represented by the quality manual and the associated procedures adequately meets the requirements of the applicable standard.

One suitable method of carrying out an adequacy audit is :

(i) To work through the relevant standard clause by clause, and to find the part of the documented system which applies. Use of a matrix of requirements, as a "checklist" is a good practice.

(ii) To work through the documented system (e.g. the quality manual) clause by clause, and see.

Which part of the standard applies.

It is common these days for the manual to contain a cross-reference list, and it is not unreasonable for an auditor to ask for one, as it would save time at this stage of an audit.

In all third party audits, and many second party audits, the next stage of the audit would be conditional upon acceptance of this first stage.

An adequacy audit should also seek to have clarified any ambiguous, unclear or conflicting statements on the grounds that if the auditor cannot understand them, the workforce probably can't either.

(b) ***Compliance audit / On-site audit :***

This is the audit, which seeks to establish the extent to which the documented system is implemented and observed by the workforce, i.e., are the people complying with the system?

(c) ***External audit :***

This is an audit that is performed by a company on its own suppliers or subcontractors. It may be an adequacy and/or a compliance audit.

(d) ***Internal audit :***

This is the most important of all audits, which requires company to look in on its own systems, procedures and activities in order to ascertain whether they are adequate and being complied with.

It provides management with information on whether or not their policies are being met, if the system is as efficient and as effective as it should be and whether changes are needed. It can provide a line of communication throughout the company and be a great motivator.

(e) ***Product / Process audit :***

This may be considered a vertical audit, i.e. looking at all the systems that went into the production of a specific end product or service. It should not be confused with an inspection of the item. Product audits have a number of applications. They are applicable to auditing specific projects or contracts and, because software is often produced on those lines, it is commonly used for software auditing. It applies when a company purchases only one product or service or when a specific product is being considered, for example on contract review.

Product audits are also a very useful method of auditing small organisations, either externally or internally, as almost every aspect of their system will be covered by such an audit.

It can be seen that this type of audit is also appropriate as a project audit, which can be an audit of a particular project within a large organisation.

Audits may be undertaken by relevant, trained members of an organisation's own staff or by hired,

Professional auditors. There are advantages in both options; the important consideration is which gives the most information.

A question often asked is whether specialist knowledge of the area of activity to be audited is required. In theory the answer is "no" because the auditor should be looking for objective evidence based on the requirements of the standard and provided by the documented system and conformity to it.

In practice some general knowledge is probably preferable to assist in the analysis of the acquired data and in the formation of a judgment. However, the auditor must be independent and not have direct responsibility in the area of any audit undertaken.

7.3 Why is Auditing Necessary ?

Quality audits are an essential element of the Quality Assurance function. The general objectives of quality audits are :

(a) To determine conformity or non-conformity of the quality system elements with specified requirements.

(b) To determine the effectiveness of the implemented quality system in meeting specified quality objectives.

(c) To afford an opportunity to improve the quality system.

(d) To provide Managers with information.

7.4 Principles of Auditing

(a) *Ethical conduct* : the foundation of professionalism.

Trust, Integrity, Confidentiality and discretion are essential to auditing.

(b) *Fair presentation* : the obligation to report truthfully and accurately.

(c) *Due professional care* : the application of diligence and judgment in auditing.

(d) *Independence* : the basis for the impartiality of the audit and objectivity of the audit conclusions.

(e) *Evidence based approach* : the rational method for reaching reliable and reproducible audit conclusions in a systematic audit process.

7.5 The Audit Life Cycle

A Quality systems audit can be broken down into four basic phases :

1. Planning
2. Conducting the audit
3. Analysis of results
4. Reports and Corrective Actions (including follow-up audits)

Until all phases have been fully completed, the audit cannot be considered to be finished The four phases may be termed the AUDIT LIFE CYCLE.

7.5.1 Planning for Audit

As per ISO 19011:2002, the definitions are :

7.5.2 Conducting Audit

Systematic, independent and documented processes for obtaining audit evidence evaluating it objectively to determine the extent to which the audit criteria are fulfilled.

7.5.3 Audit Criteria

Set of policies, procedures and requirements

7.5.4 Audit Evidence

Records, statements of fact or other information , which are relevant to the audit criteria and verifiable

7.5.5 Audit Findings

Results of the evaluation of the collected audit evidence against audit criteria.

7.5.6 Audit Conclusion

Outcome of an audit, provided by the audit team after consideration of the ai objectives and all audit findings.

7.5.7 Audit Client

Organisation or person requesting an audit.

7.5.8 Auditee

Organisation being audited.

7.5.9 Auditor

Person with competence to conduct an audit.

7.5.10 Audit Team

One or more auditors conducting an audit, supported if needed by technical experts.

7.5.11 Audit Plan

Description of the activities and arrangements for an audit.

7.5.12 Audit Scope

The scope of an audit is determined by the extent and boundaries of an audit.

7.5.13 Competence of Audit or ...

Demonstrated personal attributes and demonstrated ability to apply knowledge and skills determine the campetence of the auditors.

7.5.14 Independence of the Auditor

Auditors should be free from bias and influences, which could affect objectivity.

All persons and organisations involved with an audit should respect and support the independence and integrity of the auditors.

7.5.15 Forward and Backward Tracing

The auditor follows a logical sequence of process steps either starting at the input to the series and progressing to the output or working from the output and progressing back to the input.

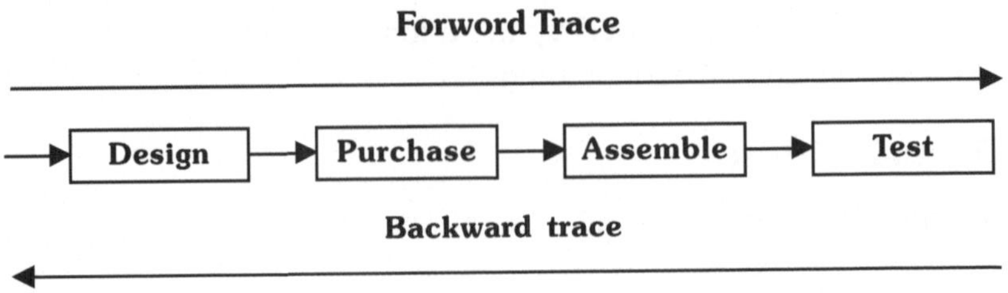

7.5.16 Trail Following

During the course of an audit, the auditor uncovers something that is worthy of further investigation, however this now leads away from the original plan of action and may even involve progressing the audit into other areas of the organisation not originally intended for audit or areas that have been/are to be audited at some other time.

WE SHOULD ALWAYS BE PREPARED TO FOLLOW TRAILS.

However sometimes it is better to take notes and follow the trail at a more convenient time or when the audit moves to the area where the trail leads.

7.5.17 Working Documents

The documents required to facilitate the auditor's investigations and to document and report results, may include :

- check Fists used for evaluating quality system elements (normally prepared by the auditor-assigned to audit that specific element);
- forms for reporting audit observations;
- forms for documenting supporting evidence for conclusions reached by the auditors.

Working documents should be designed so that they do not restrict additional audit activities or investigations which may become necessary as a result of information gathered during the audit Working documents involving confidential or proprietary information shall be suitably safeguarded by the auditing organisation.

7.5.18 Personal Attributes of Auditor

(a) ethical
(b) open minded
(c) diplomatic
(d) observant
(e) perceptive
(f) versatile
(g) tenacious
(h) decisive
(i) self-reliant

Knowledge *and* skills :

A. *General :*

(a) Audit principles, procedures, techniques

(b) Management system and reference documents
(c) Organizational situations.
(d) Applicable law, regulations, and other requirements relevant to the discipline.

B. *Specific knowledge and skills of quality management system auditors :*

(a) Quality related methods and techniques- Quality terminology, quality management principles and their application, quality management tools and their application.
(b) Process and products, including services; Sector specific terminology, technical characteristics of processes and products, including services, sector specific processes and practices.

7.6 Managing an Audit Programme

Objectives of audit programme are :

(a) Management priorities
(b) Commercial intentions
(c) Management system requirements
(d) Statutory, regulatory and contractual requirements
(e) Need for supplier evaluation
(f) Customer requirements
(g) Need for other interested parties
(h) Risks to the organisation.

7.7 Audit Methods and Techniques

These fall into three main categories each of which may be used to good effect depending upon what we are trying to achieve from the audit. However, some require more experience on the part of the auditor.

Audit methods :

Horizontal auditing

Vertical auditing

Random auditing

Each of these methods may be combined with the techniques of "forward or backward" tracing and 'trail following' to provide powerful mechanisms for verifying adequacy of implementation of Quality Systems.

7.7.1 Horizontal Auditing

Examining each functional area of an organisation to verify adequacy and implementation of Quality.

System requirements :

Used for Internal System Auditing and for Second and Third party assessments when it is necessary establish if a basic quality management system has been installed and is being implemented and maintained.

Each functional area is checked for conformance with quality system requirements, applicable to that area.

7.7.2 Vertical Auditing

Examining functional areas of an organisation that are actively contributing to a specific work package or contractual requirement

Used for contractual audit activities when a contract placing authority wishes to verify that an organisation is applying a contractually agreed quality system to all activities undertaken in support of that contract. Used extensively by Ministry of Defence and other major contract placers.

Functional areas of the organisation and interfaces with the contract placer are examined to verify conformance with contractually agreed quality system requirements, which may be detailed in a contract specific quality plan or programme.

The audit team usually works through the logical sequence of events undertaken following contract negotiation and pass through those functional areas contributing to the contract as the logical sequence is followed.

7.7.3 Random Auditing

Examinies various aspects of an organisations operation as determined by the auditor and due to the need to closely examine a particular activity or generally probe the system in a random manner.

7.8 Audit Programme Records

(a) Records related to individual audits - audit plans, audit reports, nonconformity reports, corrective and preventive action reports, audit follow up reports.

(b) Results of audit programme review.

(c) Records related to audit personnel covering subjects such as auditor competence and performance evaluation, audit team selection, maintenance and improvement of competence.

7.9 Overview of Audit Activities

The overview of all audit activities in chronological order are shown in Fig. 7.1 while that of audit activities are shown in Fig. 7.2.

Overview of typical audit activities

Initiating the audit
Appointing the audit team leader
defining audit objectives, scope, criteria
determining the feasibility of the audit
selecting the audit team
establishing initial contact with the auditee

↓

Conducting document review

Reviewing relevant management system documents, including records and determining their adequacy with respect to audit criteria.

↓

Preparing for the on-site audit activities

Preparing the audit plan
Assigning work to the audit team

↓

Conducting on-site audit activities

Conducting opening meeting
Communication during the audit
Roles and responsibilities of guides and observers
Collecting and verifying information
Generating audit findings Preparing audit conclusions

↓

Preparing, approving and distributing the audit report

Preparing the audit report
Approving and distributing the audit report

↓

Completing the audit

↓

Conducting the audit follow-up

Figure 7.1 Overview of audit activities

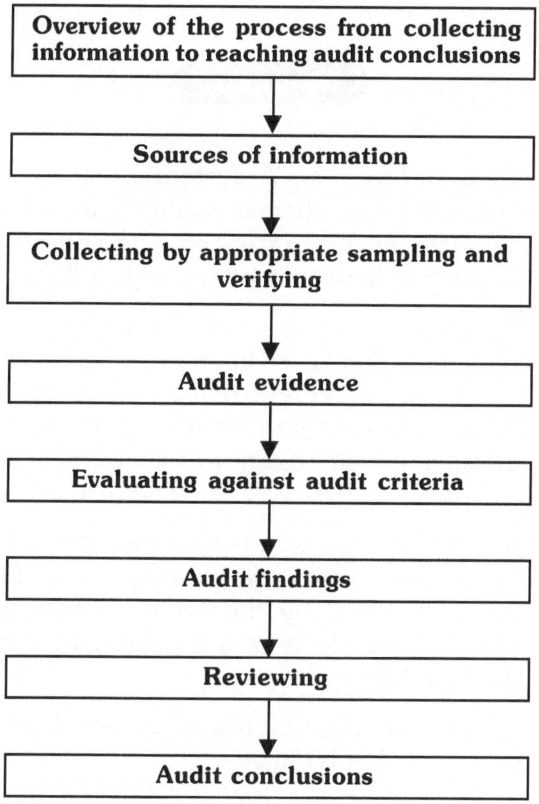

Figure 7.2 Overview of audit analysis.

Summary

Quality Audit is defined as "A systematic and independent examination to determine whether quality activities and related results comply with planned arrangements and whether these arrangements are implemented effectively and are suitable to achieve objectives

As defined then, an audit is an information gathering activity so that the need for improvement or corrective action may be evaluated. There is no element of a witch hunt or apportioning blame for problems. It is important to establish this fact amongst auditees because defensiveness is not conducive to information flow.

Audits may be internal or external and do not necessarily have to cover the whole system at once but may cover elements of it. Independence is ensured by the auditors having no direct responsibility in the audited area but preferably working in co-operation with the relevant

Audits may be undertaken by relevant, trained members of an organisation's own staff or by hired,

Quality audits are an essential element of the Quality Assurance function. The general objectives of quality audits are :

(a) To determine conformity or non-conformity of the quality system elements with specified requirements.

(b) To determine the effectiveness of the implemented quality system in meeting specified quality objectives.

(c) To afford an opportunity to improve the quality system.

(d) To provide Managers with information.

The audit life cycle :

A quality systems audit can be broken down into four basis phases:

1. Planning.
2. Conducting the audit.
3. Analysis of results.
4. Reports and corrective actions (including follow-up audits).

Questions

1. What do you mean by a quality audit? Describe in brief the outline of an audit?
2. What are the different types of audit? Explain its importance with respect to a pharmaceutical industry? Why do you feel that audit is necessary?
3. Explain what do you mean by the audit cycle?
4. What are the principles of auditing?
5. How do you conduct an audit programme ?
6. Explain in detail audit methods and techniques involved?
7. What do you mean by Forward and backward tracing, trail following?
8. What are the personal attributes of an auditor?

Appendix-I

Elements of ISO 9001, 2000

Quality Management Systems — Requirements

1 Scope

1.1 General

This International Standard specifies requirements for a quality management system where an organization.

(a) needs to demonstrate Its ability to consistently provide product that meets customer and applicable regulatory requirements, and

(b) aims to enhance customer satisfaction through the effective application of the system, including processes fur continual improvement of the system and the assurance of conformity to customer and applicable regulatory requirements.

Note : *In this International Standard, the term "product" applies only to the product intended for, or required by a customer.*

1.2 Application

All requirements of this International Standard are generic and are intended to be applicable to all organizations, regardless of type, size and product provided.

Where any requirements) of this International Standard cannot be applied due to the nature of an organization and 'is product, [his can be considered for exclusion

Where exclusions are made, claims of conformity to this International Standard are not acceptable unless these exclusions are limited to requirements within clause 7, and such exclusions do not affect the organization's ability, or responsibility, to provide product that meets customer and applicable regulatory requirements.

2 Normative References

The following normative document contains provisions which, through reference in this text, constitute provisions of this International Standard. For dated references, subsequent amendments to, or revisions of, any of these publications do not apply. However, parties to agreements based on this International Standard are encouraged investigate the possibility of applying the most recent edition of the normative document indicated below. For undated references, the latest edition of the normative document referred to applies. Members of ISO and IEC maintain registers of currently valid International Standards.

ISO 9000:2000, Quality management systems — Fundamentals and vocabulary.

3 Terms and Definitions

For the purposes of this International Standard, the terms and definitions given in ISO 9000 apply

The following terms, used in this edition of ISO 9001 to describe the supply chain, have been changed to reflect the vocabulary currently used:

supplier → organization → customer

The term "organization" replaces the term "supplier" used in ISO 9001:1994, and refers to the unit to which this International Standard applies. Also, the term "supplier" now replaces the term "subcontractor".

Throughout the text of this International Standard, wherever the term "product" occurs, it can also mean "service",

4 Quality Management System

4.1 General requirements

The organization shall establish, document, implement and maintain a quality management system and continually improve its effectiveness in accordance with the requirements of this International Standard.

The organization shall,

(a) identify the processes needed for the quality management system and their application throughout the organization,

(b) determine the sequence and interaction of these processes,

(c) determine criteria and methods needed to ensure that both the operation and control of these processes are effective,

(d) ensure the availability of resources and information necessary to support the operation and monitoring) of these processes,

(e) monitor, measure and analyse these processes, and

(f) implement actions necessary to achieve planned results and continual Improvement of these processes.

These processes shall be managed by the organization in accordance with the requirements of this International Standard.

Where an organization chooses to outsource any process that affects product conformity with requirements, the organization shall ensure control over such processes. Control of such outsourced processes shall be identified within the quality management system.

Note : Processes needed for the quality management system referred to above should include processes for management activities, provision of resources, product realization and measurement.

4.2 Documentation requirements

4.2.1 General

The quality management system documentation shall include :

(a) documented statements of a quality policy and quality objectives,

(b) a quality manual,

(c) documented procedures required by this International Standard,

(d) documents needed by the organization to ensure the effective planning, operation and control of its processes, and

(e) records required by this International Standard.

Note 1 : Where the term "documented procedure" appears within this International Standard, this means that the procedure is established, documented, implemented and maintained.

Note 2 : The extent of the quality management system documentation can differ from one organization to another due to,

(a) the size of organization and type of activities,

(b) the complexity of processes and their interactions, and

(c) the competence of personnel-

Note 3 : The documentation can be in any form or type of medium.

4.2.2 Quality Manual

The organization shall establish and maintain a quality manual that includes :

(a) the scope of the quality management system, including details of and justification for any exclusions,

(b) the documented procedures established for the quality management system, or reference to them, and

(c) a description 'of the interaction between the processes of the quality management system.

4.2.3 Control of Documents

Documents required by the quality management system shall be controlled. Records are a special type of document and shall be controlled according to the requirements given in 4.2.4.

A documented procedure shall be established to define the controls needed,

(a) to approve documents for adequacy prior to issue,

(b) to review and update as necessary and re-approve documents.

(c) to ensure that changes and the current revision status of documents are identified,

(d) to ensure that relevant versions of applicable documents are available at points of use,

(e) to ensure that documents remain legible and readily identifiable,

(f) to ensure that documents of external origin are identified and their distribution controlled, and

(g) to prevent the unintended use of obsolete documents, and to apply suitable identification to them If they are retained for any purpose.

4.2.4 Control of Records

Records shall be established and maintained to provide evidence of conformity to requirements and of the effective operation of the quality management system. Records shaft remain legible, readily identifiable and retrievable A documented procedure shall be established to define the controls needed for the identification, storage, protection, retrieval, retention time and disposition of records.

5 Management Responsibility

5.1 Management Commitment

Top management shall provide evidence of its commitment to the development and implementation of the quality management system and continually improving its effectiveness by

(a) communicating to the organization the importance of meeting customer as well as statutory and regulatory requirements.

(b) establishing the quality policy,

(c) ensuring that quality objectives are established,

(d) conducting management reviews, and

(e) ensuring the availability of resources.

5.2 Customer Focus

Top management shall ensure that customer requirements are determined and are met with the aim of enhancing customer satisfaction.

5.3 Quality Policy

Top management shall ensure that the quality policy,

(a) is appropriate to the purpose of the organization,

(b) includes a commitment to comply with requirements and continually improve the effectiveness of the quality management system,

(c) provides a framework for establishing and reviewing quality objectives,

(d) is communicated and understood within the organization, and

(e) is reviewed for continuing suitability.

5.4 Planning

5.4.1 Quality Objectives

Top management snail ensure that quality objectives, including those needed lo meel requirements for product, are established at relevant functions and levels within the organization. The quality objectives shall be measurable and consistent with the quality policy.

5.4.2 Quality Management System Planning

Top management shall ensure that

(a) the planning of the quality management system is carried out in order to meet the requirements given In 4.1, as well as the quality objectives, and

(b) the integrity of the quality management system is maintained when changes to the quality management system are planned and implemented.

5.5 Responsibility, Authority and Communication

5.5.1 Responsibility and Authority

Top management shall ensure that responsibilities and authorities are defined and communicated within the organization.

5.5.2 Management Representative

Top management shall appoint a member of management who, irrespective of other responsibilities, shall have responsibility and authority that includes

(a) ensuring that processes needed for the quality management system are established. Implemented and maintained.

(b) reporting to top management on the performance of the quality management system and any need for improvement, and

(c) ensuring the promotion of awareness of customer requirements throughout the organization.

Note : The responsibility of a management representative can include liaison with external parties on matters relating to the quality management system.

5.5.3 Internal Communication

Top management shaft ensure that appropriate communication processes are established within the organization and that communication takes place regarding the effectiveness of the quality management system.

5.6 Management Review

5.6.1 General

Top management shall review the organization's quality management system, at planned Intervals, to ensure its continuing suitability, adequacy and effectiveness. This review shall include assessing opportunities for improvement and the need for changes to the quality management system, including the quality policy and quality objectives.

Records from management reviews shall be maintained.

5.6.2 Review Input

The input to management review shall include information on,

(a) results of audits,

(b) customer feedback,

(c) process performance and product conformity.

(d) status of preventive and corrective actions.

(e) follow-up actions from previous management reviews,

(f) changes that could affect the quality management system, and

(g) recommendations for improvement.

5.6.3 Review Output

The output from the management review shall include any decisions and actions related to

(a) improvement of the effectiveness of the quality management system and its processes.

(b) improvement of product related to customer requirements, and

(c) resource needs.

6 Resource Management

6.1 Provision of Resources

The organization shall determine and provide the resources needed,

(a) to implement and maintain the quality management system and continually improve its effectiveness, and

(b) to enhance customer satisfaction by meeting customer requirements.

6.2 Human Resources

6.2.1 General

Personnel performing work affecting product quality shall be competent on the basis of appropriate education, training, skills and experience.

6.2.2 Competence, Awareness and Training

The organization shall

(a) determine the necessary competence for personnel performing work affecting product quality,

(b) provide training or take other actions to satisfy these needs,

(c) evaluate the effectiveness of the actions taken,

(d) ensure that its personnel are aware of the relevance and importance of their activities and how they contribute to the achievement of the quality objectives, and

(e) maintain appropriate records of education, training, skills and experience.

6.3 Infrastructure

The organization shall determine, provide and maintain the infrastructure needed to achieve conformity lo product requirements. Infrastructure includes, as applicable,

(a) buildings, workspace and associated utilities,

(b) process equipment (both hardware and software), and

(c) supporting services (such as transport or communication).

6.4 Work Environment

The organization shall determine and manage the work environment needed to achieve conformity to product requirements.

7 Product Realization

7.1 Planning of Product Realization

The organization shall plan and develop the processes needed for product realization. Planning of product realization shall be consistent with the requirements of the other processes of the qualify management system.

In planning product realization, the organization shall determine the following, as appropriate :

(a) quality objectives and requirements for the product;

(b) the need to establish processes, documents, and provide resources specific to the product,

(c) required verification, validation, monitoring, inspection and test activities specific to the product and the criteria for product acceptance:

(d) records needed to provide evidence that the realization processes and resulting product meet requirements.

The output of this planning shall be in a form suitable for the organization's method of operations.

Note 1 : A document specifying the processes of the quality management system (including the product realization processes) and the resources to be applied to a specific product, project or contract, can be referred to as a quality plan.

Note 2 : The organization may also apply the requirements given in 7.3 to the development of product realization processes 7.2 Customer-related processes

7.2.1 Determination of Requirements Related to the Product

The organization shall determine,

(a) requirements specified by the customer, including the requirements for delivery and post-delivery activities,

(b) requirements not stated by the customer but necessary for specified or intended use, where known,

(c) statutory and regulatory requirements related to the product, and

(d) any additional requirements determined by the organization.

7.2.2 Review of Requirements Related to the Product

The organization shall review the requirements related to the product. This review shall be conducted prior to the organization's commitment to supply a product to the customer (e.g. submission of tenders, acceptance of contracts or orders, acceptance of changes to contracts or orders) and shall ensure that

(a) product requirements are defined,

(b) contract or order requirements differing from those previously expressed are resolved, and

(c) the organization has the ability to meet the defined requirements,

Records of the results of the review and actions arising from the review shall be maintained.

Where the customer provides no documented statement of requirement, the customer requirements shall be confirmed by the organization before acceptance.

Where product requirements are changed, the organization shall ensure that relevant documents are amended and that relevant personnel are made aware of the changed requirements.

> ***Note :*** In some situations, such as internet sales, a formal review is impractical for each order. Instead the review can cover relevant product information such as catalogues or advertising material.

7.2.3 Customer Communication

The organization shall determine and implement effective arrangements for communicating with customers in relation to

(a) product information,

(b) enquiries, contracts or order handling, including amendments, and

(c) customer feedback, including customer complaints.

7.3 Design and Development

7.3.1 Design and Development Planning

The organization shall plan and control the design and development of product.

During the design and development planning, the organization shall determine,

(a) the design and development stages,

(b) the review, verification and validation that are appropriate to each design and development stage, and

(c) the responsibilities and authorities for design and development.

The organization shall manage the interfaces between different groups involved In design and development to ensure effective communication and clear assignment of responsibility-Planning output shall be updated, as appropriate, as the design and development progresses.

7.3.2 Design and Development Inputs

Inputs relating to product requirements shall be determined and records maintained. These inputs shall include,

(a) functional and performance requirements,

(b) applicable statutory and regulatory requirements,

(c) where applicable, information derived from previous similar designs, and

(d) other requirements essential for design and development.

These inputs shall be reviewed for adequacy. Requirements shall be complete, unambiguous and not in conflict with each other.

7.3.3 Design and Development Outputs

The outputs of design and development shall be provided in a form that enables verification against the design and development input and shall be approved prior to release.

Design and development outputs shall,

(a) meet the input requirements for design and development,

(b) provide appropriate information for purchasing, production and for service provision,

(c) contain or reference product acceptance criteria, and

(d) specify the characteristics of the product that are essential for its safe and proper use.

7.3.4 Design and Development Review

At suitable stages, systematic reviews of design and development shall be performed in accordance with planned arrangements.

(a) to evaluate the ability of the results of design and development to meet requirements, and

(b) to identify any problems and propose necessary actions-Participants in such reviews shall include representatives of functions concerned with the design and development stage(s) being reviewed. Records of the results of the reviews and any necessary actions shall be maintained.

7.3.5 Design and Development Verification

Verification shall be performed in accordance with planned arrangements (see 7.3.1) to ensure that the design and development outputs have met the design and development input requirements. Records of the results of the verification and any necessary actions shall be maintained.

7.3.6 Design and Development Validation

Design and development validation shall be performed in accordance with planned arrangements (see 7.3.1) to ensure that (he resulting product is capable of meeting the requirements for the specified application or intended use, where known. Wherever practicable, validation shall be completed prior to the delivery or implementation of the product. Records of the results of validation and any necessary actions shall be maintained.

7.3.7 Control of Design and Development Changes

Design and development changes shall be identified and records maintained. The changes shall be reviewed, verified and validated, as appropriate, and approved before implementation. The review of design and development changes shall include evaluation of the effect of the changes on constituent parts and product already delivered.

Records of the results of the review of changes and any necessary actions shall be maintained.

7.4 Purchasing

7.4.1 Purchasing Process

The organization shall ensure that purchased product conforms to specified purchase requirements. The type and extent of control applied to the supplier and the purchased product shall be dependent upon the effect of the purchased product on subsequent product realization or the final product.

The organization shall evaluate and select suppliers based on their ability to supply product In accordance with the organization's requirements. Criteria for selection, evaluation and re-evaluation shall be established.

Records of the results of evaluations and any necessary actions arising from the evaluation shall be maintained.

7.4.2 Purchasing Information

Purchasing information shall describe the product to be purchased, including where appropriate,

(a) requirements for approval of product, procedures, processes and equipment,

(b) requirements for qualification of personnel, and

(c) quality management system requirements.

The organization shall ensure the adequacy of specified purchase requirements prior to their communication to the supplier.

7.4.3 Verification of Purchased Product

The organization shall establish and implement the inspection or other activities necessary for ensuring that purchased product meets specified purchase requirements.

Where the organization or its customer intends to perform verification at the supplier's premises, the organization shall state the intended verification arrangements and method of product release in the purchasing information.

7.5 Production and Service Provision

7.5.1 Control of Production and Service Provision

The organization shall plan and carry out production and service provision under controlled conditions. Controlled conditions shall include, as applicable

(a) the availability of information that describes the characteristics of the product.

(b) the availability of work instructions, as necessary,

(c) the use of suitable equipment,

(d) the availability and use of monitoring and measuring devices,

(e) the implementation of monitoring and measurement, and

(f) the implementation of release, delivery and post-delivery activities.

7.5.2 Validation of Processes for Production and Service Provision

The organization shall validate any processes for production and service provision where the resulting output cannot e verified by subsequent monitoring or measurement. This includes any processes where deficiencies become apparent only after the product is in use or the service has been delivered.

Validation shall demonstrate the ability of these processes to achieve planned results.

The organization shall establish arrangements for these processes including, as applicable,

(a) defined criteria for review and approval of the processes,

(b) approval of equipment and qualification of personnel,

(c) use of specific methods and procedures,

(d) requirements for records, and

(e) revalidation.

7.5.3 Identification and Trace Ability

Where appropriate, the organization shall identity the product by suitable means throughout product realization.

The organization shall identify the product status with respect to monitoring and measurement requirements.

Where trace ability is a requirement, the organization shall control and record the unique identification of the product.

Note : In some industry sectors, configuration management is a means by which identification and trace ability are maintained.

7.5.4 Customer Property

The organization shall exercise care with customer property while it is under the organization's control or being used by the organization. The organization shall identify, verify, protect and safeguard customer property provided for use or incorporation into the product. If any customer property is lost, damaged or otherwise found to be unsuitable for use, this shall be reported to the customer and records maintained.

Note : Customer property can include intellectual property.

7.5.5 Preservation of Product

The organization shall preserve the conformity of product during internal processing and delivery to the intended destination. This preservation shall include identification, handling, packaging, storage and protection. Preservation shall also apply to the constituent parts of a product.

7.6 Control of Monitoring and Measuring Devices

The organization shall determine the monitoring and measurement to be undertaken and the monitoring and measuring devices needed to provide evidence of conformity of product to determined requirements.

The organization shall establish processes to ensure that monitoring and measurement can be carried out and are carried out in a manner that is **consistent** with the monitoring and measurement requirements.

Where necessary to ensure valid results, measuring equipment shall

(a) be calibrated or verified at specified intervals, or prior to use, against measurement standards traceable to international or national measurement standards; where no such standards exist, the basis used for calibration or verification shall be recorded;

(b) be adjusted or re-adjusted as necessary;

(c) be identified to enable the calibration status to be determined;

(d) be safeguarded from adjustments that would invalidate the measurement result;

(e) be protected from damage and deterioration during handling, maintenance and storage.

In addition, the organization shall assess and record the validity of the previous measuring results when the equipment is found not to conform to requirements. The organization shall take appropriate action on the equipment and any product affected. Records of the results of calibration and verification shall be maintained.

When used in the monitoring and measurement of specified requirements, the ability of computer software to satisfy the intended application shall be confirmed. This shall be undertaken prior to initial use and reconfirmed as necessary,

NOTE See ISO 10012-1 and ISO 10012-2 for guidance.

8 Measurement, Analysis and Improvement

8.1 General

The organization shall plan and implement the monitoring, measurement, analysis and improvement processes needed

(a) to demonstrate conformity of the product,

(b) to ensure conformity of the quality management system, and

(c) to continually improve the effectiveness of the quality management system.

This shall include determination of applicable methods, including statistical techniques, and the extent of their use.

8.2 Monitoring and Measurement

8.2.1 Customer Satisfaction

As one of the measurements of the performance of the quality management system, the organization shall monitor information relating to customer perception as to whether the organization has met customer requirements. The methods for obtaining and using this information shall be determined.

8.2.2 Internal Audit

The organization shall conduct internal audits at planned intervals to determine whether the quality management system

(a) conforms to the planned arrangements, to the requirements of this International Standard and to the quality management system requirements established by the organization, and

(b) is effectively implemented and maintained.

An audit programme shall be planned, taking into consideration the status and importance of the processes and areas to be audited as well as the results of previous audits. The audit criteria, scope, frequency and methods shall be defined. Selection of auditors and conduct of audits shall ensure objectivity and impartiality of the audit process; Auditors shall not audit their own work.

The responsibilities and requirements for planning and conducting audits, and for reporting results and maintaining records (see 4.2.4) shall be defined in a documented procedure.

The management responsible for the area being audited shall ensure that actions are taken without undue delay to eliminate detected nonconformities and their causes. Follow-up activities shall include the verification of the actions taken and the reporting of verification results.

NOTE See ISO 10011-1, ISO 10011-2 and ISO 10011-3 for guidance.

8.2.3 Monitoring and Measurement of Processes

The organization shall apply suitable methods for monitoring and, where applicable, measurement of the quality management system processes. These methods shall demonstrate the ability of the processes to achieve planned results. When planned results are not achieved, correction and corrective action shall be taken, as appropriate, to ensure conformity of the product.

8.2.4 Monitoring and Measurement of Product

The organization shall monitor and measure the characteristics of the product to verify that product requirements have been met. This shall be carried out at appropriate stages of the product realization process in accordance with the planned arrangements.

Evidence of conformity with the acceptance criteria shall be maintained. Records shall indicate the person(s) authorizing release of *product.*

Product release and service delivery shall not proceed until the planned arrangements have been satisfactorily completed, unless otherwise approved by a relevant authority and, where applicable, by the customer.

8.3 Control of Nonconforming Product

The organization shall ensure that product which does not conform to product requirements is identified and controlled to prevent its unintended use or delivery. The controls and related responsibilities and authorities for dealing with nonconforming product shall be defined in a documented procedure.

The organization shall deal with nonconforming product by one or more of the following ways;

(a) *by taking action to eliminate the detected nonconformity;*

(b) by authorizing its use, release or acceptance under concession by a relevant authority and, where applicable, by the customer,

(c) by taking action to preclude its original intended use or application.

Records of the nature of nonconformities and any subsequent actions taken, including concessions obtained, shall be maintained.

When nonconforming product is corrected it shall be subject to re-verification lo demonstrate conformity to the requirements. When nonconforming product is detected after delivery or use has started, the organization shall take action appropriate to the effects, or potential effects, of the nonconformity.

8.4 Analysis of Data

The organization shall determine, collect and analyse appropriate data to demonstrate the suitability and effectiveness of the quality management system and to evaluate where continual improvement of the effectiveness of the quality management system can be made- This shall include data generated as a result of monitoring and measurement and from other relevant sources.

The analysis of data shall provide information relating to,

(a) customer satisfaction,

(b) conformity to product requirements,

(c) characteristics and trends of processes and products including opportunities for preventive action, and

(d) suppliers.

8.5 Improvement

8.5.1 Continual Improvement

The organization shall continually improve the effectiveness of the quality management system through the use of the quality policy, quality objectives, audit results, analysis of data, corrective and preventive actions and management review.

8.5.2 Corrective Action

The organization shall take action to eliminate the cause of nonconformities in order to prevent recurrence Corrective actions shall be appropriate to the effects of the nonconformities encountered

A documented procedure shall be established to define requirements for

(a) reviewing nonconformities (including customer complaints),

(b) determining (he causes of nonconformities,

(c) evaluating the need for action to ensure that nonconformities do not recur,

(d) determining and implementing action needed,

(e) records of the results of action taken and

(f) reviewing corrective action taken.

8.5.3 Preventive Action

The organization shall determine action to eliminate the causes of potential nonconformities in order to prevent their occurrence. Preventive actions shall be appropriate to the effects of the potential problems.

1 Quality Management System

1.1 General Requirements

The organization shall establish, documents, implement, maintain and continually improve a quality management system in accordance with the requirements of this international standard.

The organization shall :

(a) Identify the processes needed for the quality managements system and their application throughout the organization.

(b) Determine the sequence and interaction of these processes.

(c) Determine criteria and methods needed to ensure that both the operation and control of these processes are effective.

(d) Ensure the availability of resources and information necessary to support the operation and monitoring of these processes.

(e) Monitor, measure and analyze these processes, and

(f) Implement action necessary to achieve planned results and continual improvement of these processes.

These processes shall be managed by the organization in accordance with requirements of this international Standard.

Where an organization chooses to outsource any process that affects product conformity with requirements, the organization shall ensure control over such processes. Control of such outsourced processes shall be identified within the quality management system.

Note : Processes needed for the quality management system referred to above should include processes for management activities, provision of resources, product realization and measurement.

1.2 Documentation Requirements

1.2.1 General

The quality management system documentation shall include

(a) Documented statements of a quality policy and quality objectives.

(b) A quality manual.

(c) Documented procedures required by this international standard;

(d) Documents needed by the organization to ensure the effective planning, operation and control of its processes, and

(e) Records required by this international standard

Note 1 : Where the term-documented procedure appears within this international standard, this means that the procedure is established, documented, implemented and maintained.

Note 2 : The extent of the quality management system documentation can differ from one organization to another due to :

(a) the size of the organization and type of activities,

(b) the complexity of processes and their interactions, and

(c) the competence of personnel.

Note : The documentation can be in any form or type of medium.

1.2.2 Quality Manual

The organization shall establish and maintain a quality manual that includes

(a) the scope of the quality management system, including details of the justification for the any exclusions

(b) the documented procedures established for the quality managements system, or reference to them, and

(c) a description of the interaction between the processes of the quality management system.

1.2.3 Control of Documents

Documents required by the quality management system shall be controlled. Records are a special type of documented and shall be controlled according to the requiremetns given in 1.2.4.

A documented procedure shall be established to define the controls needed.

(a) to approve documents for adequacy prior to issue,

(b) to review and update as necessary and re-approve documents

(c) to ensure that changes and the current revision status of documents are identified,

(d) to ensure that relevant versions of applicable documents are available at points of use,

(e) to ensure that documents remain legible and readily identifiable,

(f) to ensure that documents of external origin are identified and their disterubutai0on controlled, and

g) to prevent the unintended use of obsolete documents, and to apply suitable identification to them if they are retained for any purpose.

1.2.4 Control of Quality Records

Records shall be established and maintained to provide evidence of conformity to requirements and of the effective operation of the quality management system. Records shall remain legible, readily identifiable and retrievable. A documented procedure shall be established to define the controls needed for the identification, storage, protection, retrieval, retention time and disposition of records.

2 Management Responsibility

2.1 Management Commitment

Top management shall provide evidence of its commitment to the development and improvement of the quality management system and continually improving its effectiveness by

(a) communicating to the organization the importance of meeting customer as well as statutory and regulatory requirements.

(b) Establishing the quality policy,

(c) Ensuring that quality objectives are established,

(d) Conducting management reviews, and

(e) Ensuring the availability of resources

2.2 Customer Focus

Top management shall ensure that customer requirements are determined and are met with the aim of enhancing customer satisfaction.

2.3 Quality Policy

Top management shall ensure that the quality policy

(a) is appropriate to the purpose of the organization,

(b) includes a commitment to comply with requirements and continually improve the effectiveness of the quality management system

(c) provides a framework for establishing and reviewing quality objectives,

(d) is communicated and understood within the organization, and

(e) is reviewed for continuing suitability.

2.4 Planning

2.4.1 Quality objectives

Top management shall ensure that quality objectives, including those needed to meet requirements for products are established at relevant functions and levels within the organization. The quality objectives shall be measurable and consistent with the quality policy.

2.4.2 Quality Management System Planning

Top management shall ensure that

(a) the planning o the quality management system is carried out in order to meet and the requirements given in 1.1 as well as the quality objectives, and

(b) the integrity of the quality management system is maintained when changes to the quality management system are planned and implemented

2.5 Responsibility, Authority and Communication

2.5.1 Responsibility and Authority

Top management shall ensure that responsibilities and authorities are defined and communicated within the organization.

2.5.2 Management Representative

Top management shall appoint a member of the management who, irrespective of other responsibilities, shall have responsibility and authority that includes

(a) Ensuring that processes needed for the quality management system are established, implemented and maintained,

(b) Reporting to toop management on the performance of the quality management sytem and any need for improvement, and

(c) Ensuring the promotion of awareness of customer requirements throughout the organization.

Note : The responsibility of a management representative can include liaison with external parties on matters relating to the quality management system

2.5.3 Internal Communication

Top management shall ensure that appropriate communication processes are established within the organization and that communication takes place regarding the effectiveness of the quality management system.

2.6 Management Review

2.6.1 General

Top management shall review the organization's quality management system, at planned intervals, to ensure its continuing suitability, adequacy and effectiveness. This review shall include assessing opportunities for improvement and the need for changes to the quality management system including the quality policy and quality objectives.

Records from management reviews shall be maintained.

2.6.2 Review Input

The input to management review shall include information on

(a) results of audits,

(b) customer feedback,

(c) process performance and product conformity,
(d) status of preventive and corrective actions,
(e) follow-up actions from previous management reviews,
(f) changes that could affect the quality management system, and
(g) recommendations for improvement

2.6.3 Review Output

The out put from the management review shall include any decisions and actions related to

(a) improvement of the effectiveness of the quality management system and its processes,
(b) improvement of product related to customer requirements, and
(c) resource needs.

3 Resource Management

3.1 Provision of Resources

The organization shall determine and provide the resources needed

(a) to implement and maintain the quality management system and continually improve its effectiveness, and
(b) to enhance customer satisfaction by meeting customer requirements.

3.2 Human Resources

3.2.1 General

Personnel performing work affecting product quality shall be competent on the basis of appropriate education, training, skills and experience.

3.2.2 Competence, Awareness and Training

The organization shall

(a) determine the necessary competence for personnel performing work affecting product quality,

(b) provide training or take other actions to satisfy these needs,

(c) evaluate the effectiveness of actions taken,

(d) ensure that its personnel are aware of the relevance and importance of their activities and how they contribute to the achievement of the quality objectives, and

(e) maintain appropriate records of education, training, skills and experience.

3.3 Infrastructure

The organization shall determine, provide and maintain the infrastructure needed to achieve the conformity to product requirements. Infrastructure includes, as applicable,

(a) buildings, workspace and associated utilities,

(b) process equipment (both hardware and software), and

(c) supporting service (such as transport or communication).

3.4 Work Environment

The organization shall determine and mange the work environment needed to achieve conformity to product requirements.

4 Product Realization

4.1 Planning of Realization Processes

The organization shall plan and develop the processes needed for product realization. Planning or product realization shall be consistent with requirements of the other processes of the quality management system.

In planning product realization, the organization shall determine the following, as appropriate :

(a) quality objectives and requirements for the product;

(b) the need to establish processes, documents, and provide resources specific to the product;

(c) required verification, validation, monitoring, inspection and test activities specific to the product and the criteria for product acceptance;

(d) records needed to provide evidence that the realization processes and resulting product meet requirements.

The out put of this planning shall be in a form suitable for the organizations method of operations.

Note 1 **:** A document specifying the processes of the quality management system (including the product realization processes) and the resources to be applied to a specific product, project or contract can be referred to as a quality plan.

Note 2 **:** The organization may also apply the requirements given in 4.3 to the development of the product realization process.

4.2 Customer-Related Processes

4.2.1 Determination of Requirements Related to a Product

The organization shall determine

(a) requirements specified by the customer, including the requirements for delivery and post-delivery activities,

(b) requirements not stated by the customer but necessary for specific or intended use, where known,

(c) statutory and regulatory requirements related to the product, and

Records of the results of the review and actions arising from the review shall be maintained.

Where the customer provides no documented statement of requirement, the customer requirements shall be confirmed by the organization before acceptance.

Where product requirements are changed, the organization shall ensure that relevant documents are amended and that relevant personnel are made aware of the change requirements.

Note **:** In some situations, such as Internet sales, a formal review is impractical for each order. Instead the review can cover relevant product information such as catalogues or advertising material.

4.2.3 Customer Communication

The organization shall determine and implement effective arrangements for communicating with customers in relation to:

(a) product information,

(b) enquiries, contracts, or order handling, including amendments, and

(c) customer feedback, including customer complaints.

5 Measurement, Analysis and Improvement

5.1 General

The organization shall plan and implement the monitoring, measurement, analysis and improvement processes needed

(a) to demonstrate conformity of the product.

(b) To ensure conformity of the quality management system, and

(c) To continually improve the effectiveness of the quality management system.

This shall include the determination of applicable methods, including statistical techniques, and the extent of their use.

5.2 Monitoring and Measurement

5.2.1 Customer Satisfaction

As one of the measurements of the performance of the quality management system, the organization shall monitor information relating to customer perception as to whether the organization has met customer requirements. The methods for obtaining and using this information shall be determined.

5.2.2 Internal Audit

The organization shall conduct internal audits at planned intervals to determine whether the quality management system

(a) conforms to the planned arrangements to the requirements of this international Standard and to the quality management system requirements established by the organization, and

(b) is effectively implemented and maintained.

An audit program shall be planned, taking into consideration the status and importance of the processes and areas to be audited, as well as the results of previous audits. The audit criteria, scope, frequency and methods shall be defined. Selection of auditors and conduct of audits shall ensure objectivity and impartiality of the audit process. Auditors shall not audit their own work.

The responsibilities and requirements for planning and conducting audits, and for reporting results and maintaining records shall be defined in a documented procedure.

The management responsible for the area being audited shall ensure that the actions are taken without undue delay to eliminate detected nonconformities and their causes. Follow-up activities shall include the verification of the actions taken and the reporting of verification results.

5.2.3 Monitoring and Measurement of Processes

The organization shall apply suitable methods for monitoring and, where applicable, measurement of the quality management system processes. These methods shall demonstrate the ability of the processes to achieve planned results. When planned results are not achieved, correction and corrective action shall be taken, as appropriate, to ensure conformity of the product.

5.2.4 Monitoring and Measurement of Product

The organization shall monitor and measure the characteristics of the product to very that product requirements have been met. This shall be carried out at appropriate stages of the product realization process in accordance with the planned arrangements.

Evidence of conformity with the acceptance criteria shall be maintained. Records shall indicate the persons authorizing release of product.

Product release and service delivery shall not proceed until all the planned arrangements have been satisfactorily completed, unless otherwise approved by a relevant authority, and where applicable, by the customer.

5.3 Control of Nonconforming Product

The organization shall ensure that product which does not conform to product requirements is identified and controlled to prevent its unintended use or delivery. The controls and related responsibilities and authorities for dealing with nonconforming product shall be defined in a documented procedure.

The organization shall deal with nonconforming product by one or more of the following ways:

(a) by taking action to eliminate the detected nonconformity.

(b) by authorizing its use, release or acceptance under concession by a relevant authority and , where applicable, by the customer.

(c) by taking action to preclude its original intended use or application.

Records of the nature of nonconformities and any subsequent actions then, including concessions obtained, shall be maintained

When nonconforming product is corrected it shall be subject to re-verification to demonstrate conformity to the requirements.

When nonconforming product is detected after delivery or use has started, the organization shall take action appropriate to the effects, or potential effects, of the nonconformity.

5.4 Analysis of Data

The organization shall determine, collect and analyze appropriate date to demonstrate the suitability and effectiveness of the quality management system and to evaluate where continual improvement of the effectiveness of the quality management system can be made. This shall include data generated as a result of monitoring and measuring and from other relevant sources.

The analysis of data shall provide information relating to :

(a) customer satisfaction,

(b) conformity to product requirements,

(c) characteristics and trends of processes and products including opportunities for preventive action, and

(d) suppliers.

5.5 Improvement

5.5.1 Continual Improvement

The organization shall continually improve the effectiveness of the quality management system through the use of the quality policy, quality objectives, audit results, analysis of data, corrective and preventive actions and management review.

5.5.2 Corrective Action

The organization shall take action to eliminate the cause of nonconformities in order to prevent recurrence. Corrective action shall be appropriate to the effects of the nonconformities encountered.

A documented procedure shall be established to define requirements for

(a) reviewing nonconformities (including customer complaints).

(b) determining the causes of nonconformities,

(c) evaluating the need for action to ensure that nonconformities do not recur,

(d) determining and implementing action needed,

(e) records of the results of action taken and

(f) reviewing corrective action taken.

5.5.3 Preventive Action

The organization shall determine action to eliminate the causes of potential nonconformities in order to prevent their occurrence. Preventive actions shall be appropriate to the effects of the potential problems.

A documented procedure for preventive action shall be established to define requirements for

(a) determining potential nonconformities and their causes,

(b) evaluating the need for action to prevent occurrence of nonconformities,

(c) determining and implementing action needed,

(d) records of results of action taken and reviewing preventive action taken.

Appendix-II

Title 21 Code of Federal Regulations

Chapter 1

Food and Drug Administration Department of Health and Human Services 4-1-97 Edition

Subchapter A, Part 58

Good Laboratory Practice for Nonclinical Laboratory Studies

Subpart A - General Provisions

Sec.

58.1 Scope.

58.3 Definitions.

58.10 Applicability to studies performed under grants and contracts.

58.15 Inspection of a testing facility.

Subpart B - Organization and Personnel

58.29 Personnel.

58.31 Testing facility management.

58.33 Study director.

58.35 Quality assurance unit.

Subpart C - Facilities

58.41 General.

58.43 Animal care facilities.

58.45 Animal supply facilities.

58.47 Facilities for handling test and control articles.

58.49 Laboratory operation areas.

58.51 Specimen and data storage facilities.

Subpart D - Equipment

58.61 Equipment design.

58.63 Maintenance and calibration of equipment.

Subpart E - Testing Facilities Operation

58.81 Standard operating procedures.

58.83 Reagents and solutions.

58.90 Animal care.

Subpart F - Test and Control Articles

58.105 Test and control article characterization.

58.107 Test and control article handling.

58.113 Mixture of articles with carriers.

Subpart G - Protocol for and Conduct of a Nonclinical Laboratory Study

58.120 Protocol.

58.130 Conduct of a nonclinical laboratory study.

Subparts H - I - [Reserved]

Subpart J - Records and Reports

58.185 Reporting of nonclinical laboratory study results.

58.190 Storage and retrieval of records and data.

58.195 Retention of records.

Subpart K - Disqualification of Testing Facilities

58.200 Purpose.

58.202 Grounds for disqualification.

58.204 Notice of and opportunity for hearing or proposed disqualification.

58.206 Final order on disqualification.

58.210 Actions upon disqualification.

58.213 Public disclosure of information regarding disqualification.

58.215 Alternative or additional actions to disqualification.

58.217 Suspension or termination of a testing facility by a sponsor.

58.219 Reinstatement of a disqualified testing facility.

Authority : Secs. 402, 406, 408, 409, 501, 502, 503, 505, 506, 507, 510, 512-516, 518-520, 701, 721, 801 of the Federal Food, Drug, and Cosmetic Act (21 U.S.C. 342, 346, 346a, 348, 351, 352, 353, 355, 356, 357, 360, 360b-360f, 360h-360j, 371, 379e, 381); secs. 215, 351, 354-360F of the Public Health Service Act (42 U.S.C. 216, 262, 263b-263n).

Source : 43 FR 60013, Dec. 22, 1978, unless otherwise noted.

Subpart A - General Provisions

Sec. 58.1 Scope

(a) This part prescribes good laboratory practices for conducting nonclinical laboratory studies that support or are intended to support applications for research or marketing permits for products regulated by the Food and Drug Administration, including food and color additives, animal food additives, human and animal drugs, medical devices for human use, biological products, and electronic products. Compliance with this part is intended to assure the quality and integrity of the safety data filed pursuant to sections 406, 408, 409, 502, 503, 505, 506, 507, 510, 512-516, 518-520, 721, and 801 of the Federal Food, Drug, and Cosmetic Act and sections 351 and 354-360F of the Public Health Service Act.

(b) References in this part to regulatory sections of the Code of Federal Regulations are to Capter I of Title 21, unless otherwise noted.

[43 FR 60013, Dec. 22, 1978, as amended at 52 FR 33779, Sept. 4, 1987]

Sec. 58.3 Definitions

As used in this part, the following terms shall have the meanings specified:

(a) ***Act*** means the Federal Food, Drug, and Cosmetic Act, as amended (secs. 201-902, 52 Stat. 1040 et seq., as amended (21 U.S.C. 321-392)).

(b) ***Test article*** means any food additive, color additive, drug, biological product, electronic product, medical device for human use, or any other article subject to regulation under the act or under sections 351 and 354-360F of the Public Health Service Act.

(c) ***Control article*** means any food additive, color additive, drug, biological product, electronic product, medical device for human use, or any article other than a test article, feed, or water that is administered to the test system in the course of a nonclinical laboratory study for the purpose of establishing a basis for comparison with the test article.

(d) ***Nonclinical laboratory study*** means in vivo or in vitro experiments in which test articles are studied prospectively in test systems under laboratory conditions to determine their safety. The term does not include studies utilizing human subjects or clinical studies or field trials in animals. The term does not include basic exploratory studies carried out to determine whether a test article has any potential utility or to determine physical or chemical characteristics of a test article.

(e) ***Application for research or marketing permit includes :***

1. A color additive petition, described in part 71.
2. A food additive petition, described in parts 171 and 571.
3. Data and information regarding a substance submitted as part of the procedures for establishing that a substance is generally recognized as safe for use, which use results or may reasonably be expected to result, directly or indirectly, in its becoming a component or otherwise affecting the characteristics of any food, described in Sec. 170.35 and 570.35.

4. Data and information regarding a food additive submitted as part of the procedurres regarding food additives permitted to be used on an interim basis pending additional study, described in Sec. 180.1.
5. An investigational new drug application, described in part 312 of this chapter.
6. A new drug application, described in part 314.
7. Data and information regarding an over-the-counter drug for human use, submitted as part of the procedures for classifying such drugs as generally recognized as safe and effective and not misbranded, described in part 330.
8. Data and information about a substance submitted as part of the procedures for establishing a tolerance for unavoidable contaminants in food and food-packaging materials, described in parts 109 and 509.
9. Data and information regarding an antibiotic drug submitted as part of the procedures for issuing, amending, or repealing regulations for such drugs, described in Sec. 314.300 of this chapter.
10. A Notice of Claimed Investigational Exemption for a New Animal Drug, described in part 511.
11. A new animal drug application, described in part 514.
12. [Reserved]
13. An application for a biological product license, described in part 601.
14. An application for an investigational device exemption, described in part 812.
15. An Application for Premarket Approval of a Medical Device, described in section 515 of the act.
16. A Product Development Protocol for a Medical Device, described in section 515 of the act.
17. Data and information regarding a medical device submitted as part of the procedures for classifying such devices, described in part 860.
18. Data and information regarding a medical device submitted as part of the procedures for establishing, amending, or repealing a performance standard for such devices, described in part 861.

19. Data and information regarding an electronic product submitted as part of the procedures for obtaining an exemption from notification of a radiation safety defect of failure of compliance with a radiation safety performance standard, described in subpart D of part 1003.
20. Data and information regarding an electronic product submitted as part of the procedures for establishing, amending, or repealing a standard for such product, described in section 358 of the Public Health Service Act.
21. Data and information regarding an electronic product submitted as part of the procedures for obtaining a variance from any electronic product performance standard as described in Sec. 1010.4.
22. Data and information regarding an electronic product submitted as part of the procedures for granting, amending, or extending an exemption from any electronic product performance standard, as described in Sec. 1010.5.

(f) ***Sponsor means :***

1. A person who initiates and supports, by provision of financial or other resources, a nonclinical laboratory study;
2. A person who submits a nonclinical study to the Food and Drug Administration in support of an application for a research or marketing permit; or
3. A testing facility, if it both initiates and actually conducts the study.

(g) ***Testing facility*** means a person who actually conducts a nonclinical laboratory study, i.e., actually uses the test article in a test system. *Testing facility* includes any establishment required to register under section 510 of the act that conducts nonclinical laboratory studies and any consulting laboratory described in section 704 of the act that conducts such studies. *Testing facility* encompasses only those operational units that are being or have been used to conduct nonclinical laboratory studies.

(h) ***Person includes*** an individual, partnership, corporation, association, scientific or academic establishment, government agency, or organizational unit thereof, and any other legal entity.

(i) ***Test system*** means any animal, plant, microorganism, or subparts thereof to which the test or control article is administered or added for study. *Test system* also includes appropriate groups or components of the system not treated with the test or control articles.

(j) ***Specimen*** means any material derived from a test system for examination or analysis.

(k) ***Raw data*** means any laboratory worksheets, records, memoranda, notes, or exact copies thereof, that are the result of original observations and activities of a nonclinical laboratory study and are necessary for the reconstruction and evaluation of the report of that study. In the event that exact transcripts of raw data have been prepared (e.g., tapes which have been transcribed verbatim, dated, and verified accurate by signature), the exact copy or exact transcript may be substituted for the original source as raw data. *Raw data* may include photographs, microfilm or microfiche copies, computer printouts, magnetic media, including dictated observations, and recorded data from automated instruments.

(l) ***Quality assurance unit*** means any person or organizational element, except the study director, designated by testing facility management to perform the duties relating to quality assurance of nonclinical laboratory studies.

(m) ***Study director*** means the individual responsible for the overall conduct of a nonclinical laboratory study.

(n) *Batch means* a specific quantity or lot of a test or control article that has been characterized according to Sec. 58.105(a).

(o) ***Study initiation date*** means the date the protocol is signed by the study director.

(p) ***Study completion date*** means the date the final report is signed by the study director.

[43 FR 60013, Dec. 22. 1978, as amended at 52 FR 33779, Sept. 4, 1987; 54 FR 9039, Mar. 3,1989]

Sec. 58.10 Applicability to studies performed under grants and contracts

When a sponsor conducting a nonclinical laboratory study intended to be submitted to or reviewed by the Food and Drug Administration utilizes the services of a consulting laboratory, contractor, or grantee to perform an analysis or other service, it shall notify the consulting laboratory, contractor, or grantee that the service is part of a nonclinical laboratory study that must be conducted in compliance with the provisions of this part.

Sec. 58.15 Inspection of a testing facility

(a) A testing facility shall permit an authorized employee of the Food and Drug Administration, at reasonable times and in a reasonable manner, to inspect the facility and to inspect (and in the case of records also to copy) all records and specimens required to be maintained regarding studies within the scope of this part. The records inspection and copying requirements shall not apply to quality assurance unit records of findings and problems, or to actions recommended and taken.

(b) The Food and Drug Administration will not consider a nonclinical laboratory study in support of an application for a research or marketing permit if the testing facility refuses to permit inspection. The determination that a nonclinical laboratory study will not be considered in support of an application for a research or marketing permit does not, however, relieve the applicant for such a permit of any obligation under any applicable statute or regulation to submit the results of the study to the Food and Drug Administration.

Subpart B - Organization and Personnel

Sec. 58.29 Personnel

(a) Each individual engaged in the conduct of or responsible for the supervision of a nonclinical laboratory study shall have education, training, and experience, or combination thereof, to enable that individual to perform the assigned functions.

(b) Each testing facility shall maintain a current summary of training and experience and job description for each individual engaged in or supervising the conduct of a nonclinical laboratory study.

(c) There shall be a sufficient number of personnel for the timely and proper conduct of the study according to the protocol.

(d) Personnel shall take necessary personal sanitation and health precautions designed to avoid contamination of test and control articles and test systems.

(e) Personnel engaged in a nonclinical laboratory study shall wear clothing appropriate for the duties they perform. Such clothing shall be changed as often as necessary to prevent microbiological, radiological, or chemical contamination of test systems and test and control articles.

(f) Any individual found at any time to have an illness that may adversely affect the quality and integrity of the nonclinical laboratory study shall be excluded from direct contact with test systems, test and control articles and any other operation or function that may adversely affect the study until the condition is corrected. All personnel shall be instructed to report to their immediate supervisors any health or medical conditions that may reasonably be considered to have anadverse effect on a nonclinical laboratory study.

Sec. 58.31 Testing facility management

For each nonclinical laboratory study, testing facility management shall:

(a) Designate a study director as described in Sec. 58.33, before the study is initiated.

(b) Replace the study director promptly if it becomes necessary to do so during the conduct of a study.

(c) Assure that there is a quality assurance unit as described in Sec. 58.35.

(d) Assure that test and control articles or mixtures have been appropriately tested for identity, strength, purity, stability, and uniformity, as applicable.

(e) Assure that personnel, resources, facilities, equipment, materials, and methodologies are available as scheduled.

(f) Assure that personnel clearly understand the functions they are to perform.

(g) Assure that any deviations from these regulations reported by the quality assurance unit are communicated to the study director and corrective actions are taken and documented.

[43 FR 60013, Dee. 22, 1978, as amended at 52 FR 33780, Sept. 4, 1987]

Sec. 58.33 Study director

For each nonclinical laboratory study, a scientist or other professional of appropriate education, training, and experience, or combination thereof, shall be identified as the study director. The study director has overall responsibility for the technical conduct of the study, as well as for the interpretation, analysis, documentation and reporting of results, and represents the single point of study control. The study director shall assure that :

(a) The protocol, including any change, is approved as provided by Sec. 58.120 and is followed.

(b) All experimental data, including observations of unanticipated responses of the test system are accurately recorded and verified.

(c) Unforeseen circumstances that may affect the quality and integrity of the nonclinical laboratory study are noted when they occur, and corrective action is taken and documented.

(d) Test systems are as specified in the protocol.

(e) All applicable good laboratory practice regulations are followed.

(f) All raw data, documentation, protocols, specimens, and final reports are transferred to the archives during or at the close of the study.

[43 FR 60013, Dec. 22, 1978; 44 FR 17657, Mar. 23, 1979]

Sec. 58.35 Quality assurance unit

(a) A testing facility shall have a quality assurance unit which shall be responsible for monitoring each study to assure management that the facilities, equipment, personnel, methods, practices, records, and controls are In conformance with the regulations in this part. For any given study, the quality assurance unit shall be entirely separate from and independent of the personnel engaged in the direction and conduct of that study.

(b) The quality assurance unit shall :

1. Maintain a copy of a master schedule sheet of all nonclinical laboratory studies conducted at the testing facility indexed by test article and containing the test system, nature of study, date study was initiated, current status of each study, identity of the sponsor, and name of the study director.
2. Maintain copies of all protocols pertaining to all nonclinical laboratory studies for which the unit is responsible.

3. Inspect each nonclinical laboratory study at intervals adequate to assure the integrity of the study and maintain written and properly signed records of each periodic inspection showing the date of the inspection, the study inspected, the phase or segment of the study inspected, the person performing the inspection, findings and problems, action recommended and taken to resolve existing problems, and any scheduled date for reinspection. Any problems found during the course of an inspection which are likely to affect study integrity shall be brought to the attention of the study director and management immediately.
4. Periodically submit to management and the study director written status reports on each study, noting any problems and the corrective actions taken.
5. Determine that no deviations from approved protocols or standard operating procedures were made without proper authorization and documentation.
6. Review the final study report to assure that such report accurately describes the methods and standard operating procedures, and that the reported results accurately reflect the raw data of the nonclinical laboratory study.
7. Prepare and sign a statement to be included with the final study report which shall specify the dates inspections were made and findings reported to management and to the study director.

(c) The responsibilities and procedures applicable to the quality assurance unit, the records maintained by the quality assurance unit, and the method of indexing such records shall be in writing and shall be maintained. These items Including inspection dates, the study inspected, the phase or segment of the study inspected, and the name of the individual performing the inspection shall be made available for inspection to authorized employees of the Food and Drug Administration.

(d) A designated representative of the Food and Drug Administration shall have access to the written procedures established for the inspection and may request testing facility management to certify that inspections are being implemented, performed, documented, and followed-up in accordance with this paragraph.

(Information collection requirements approved by the Office of Management and Budget under control number 0910-0203)

[43 FR 60013, Dec. 22, 1978, as amended at 52 FR 33780, Sept. 4, 1987]

Subpart C - Facilities

Sec. 58.41 General.

Each testing facility shall be of suitable size and construction to facilitate the proper conduct of nonclinical laboratory studies. It shall be designed so that there is a degree of separation that will prevent any function or activity from having in adverse effect on the study.

[52 FR 33780, Sept. 4, 1987]

SS 58.43 Animal care facilities

(a) A testing facility shall have a sufficient number of animal rooms or areas, as needed, to assure proper : 1. Separation of species or test systems, 2. isolation of individual projects, 3. quarantine of animals, and 4. routine or specialized housing of animals.

(b) A testing facility shall have a number of animal rooms or areas separate from those described in paragraph (a) of this section to ensure isolation of studies being done with test systems or test and control articles known to be biohazardous, including volatile substances, aerosols, radioactive materials, and infectious agents.

(c) Separate areas shall be provided, as appropriate, for the diagnosis, treatment, and control of laboratory animal diseases. These areas shall provide effective isolation for the housing of animals either known or suspected of being diseased, or of being carriers of disease, from other animals.

(d) When animals are housed, facilities shall exist for the collection and disposal of all animal waste and refuse or for safe sanitary storage of waste before removal from the testing facility. Disposal facilities shall be so provided and operated as to minimize vermin infestation, odors, disease hazards, and environmental contamination.

[43 FR 60013, Dec. 22, 1978, as amended at 52 FR 33780, Sept. 4, 1987]

Sec. 58.45 Animal supply facilities

There shall be storage areas, as needed, for feed, bedding, supplies, and equipment. Storage areas for feed and bedding shall be separated from areas housing the test systems and shall be protected against infestation or contamination. Perishable supplies shall be preserved by appropriate means.

[43 FR 60013, Dec. 22, 1978, as amended at 52 FR 33780, Sept. 4, 1987]

Sec. 58.47 Facilities for handling test and control articles

(a) As necessary to prevent contamination or mixups, there shall be separate areas for :

1. Receipt and storage of the test and control articles.
2. Mixing of the test and control articles with a carrier, e.g., feed.
3. Storage of the test and control article mixtures.

(b) Storage areas for the test and/or control article and test and control mixtures shall be separate from areas housing the test systems and shall be adequate to preserve the identity, strength, purity, and stability of the articles and mixtures.

Sec. 58.49 Laboratory operation areas

Separate laboratory space shall be provided, as needed, for the performance of the routine and specialized procedures required by nonclinical laboratory studies.

[52 FR 33780, Sept. 4, 1987]

Sec. 58.51 Specimen and data storage facilities

Space shall be provided for archives, limited to access by authorized personnel only, for the storage and retrieval of all raw data and specimens from completed studies.

Subpart D - Equipment

Sec. 58.61 Equipment design

Equipment used in the generation, measurement, or assessment of data and equipment used for facility environmental control shall be of appropriate design and adequate capacity to function according to the protocol and shall be suitably located for operation, inspection, cleaning, and maintenance.

[52 FR 33780, Sept. 4, 1987]

Sec. 58.63 Maintenance and calibration of equipment

(a) Equipment shall be adequately inspected, cleaned, and maintained. Equipment used for the generation, measurement, or assessment of data shall be adequately tested, calibrated and/or standardized.

(b) The written standard operating procedures required under Sec. 58.81(b)(11) shall set forth in sufficient detail the methods, materials, and schedules to be used in the routine inspection, cleaning, maintenance, testing, calibration, and/or standardization of equipment, and shall specify, when appropriate, remedial action to be taken in the event of failure or malfunction of equipment. The written standard operating procedures shall designate the person responsible for the performance of each operation.

(c) Written records shall be maintained of all inspection, maintenance, testing, calibrating and/or standardizing operations. These records, containing the date of the operation, shall describe whether the maintenance operations were routine and followed the written standard operating procedures. Written records shall be kept of nonroutine repairs performed on equipment as a result of failure and malfunction. Such records shall document the nature of the defect, how and when the defect was discovered, and any remedial action taken in response to the defect.

(Information collection requirements approved by the Office of Management and Budget under control number 0910-0203)

[43 FR 60013, Dec. 22, 1978, as amended at 52 FR 33780, Sept. 4, 1987]

Subpart E - Testing Facilities Operation

Sec. 58.81 Standard operating procedures

(a) A testing facility shall have standard operating procedures in writing setting forth nonclinical laboratory study methods that management is satisfied are adequate to insure the quality and integrity of the data generated in the course of a study. All deviations in a study from standard operating procedures shall be authorized by the study director and shall be documented in the raw data. Significant changes in established standard operating procedures shall be properly authorized in writing by management.

(b) Standard operating procedures shall be established for, but not limited to, the following :

1. Animal room preparation.
2. Animal care.
3. Receipt, identification, storage, handling, mixing, and method of sampling of the test and control articles.

4. Test system observations.
5. Laboratory tests.
6. Handling of animals found moribund or dead during study.
7. Necropsy of animals or postmortem examination of animals.
8. Collection and identification of specimens.
9. Histopathology.
10. Data handling, storage, and retrieval.
11. Maintenance and calibration of equipment.
12. Transfer, proper placement, and identification of animals.

(c) Each laboratory area shall have immediately available laboratory manuals and standard operating procedures relative to the laboratory procedures being performed. Published literature may be used as a supplement to standard operating procedures.

(d) A historical file of standard operating procedures, and all revisions thereof, including the dates of such revisions, shall be maintained.

[43 FR 60013, Dec. 22, 1978, as amended at 52 FR 33780, Sept. 4, 1987]

Sec. 58.83 Reagents and solutions

All reagents and solutions in the laboratory areas shall be labeled to indicate Identity, titer or concentration, storage requirements, and expiration date. Deteriorated or outdated reagents and solutions shall not be used.

Sec. 58.90 Animal care.

(a) There shall be standard operating procedures for the housing, feeding, handling, and care of animals.

(b) All newly received animals from outside sources shall be isolated and their health status shall be evaluated in accordance with acceptable veterinary medical practice.

(c) At the initiation of a nonclinical laboratory study, animals shall be free of any disease or condition that might interfere with the purpose or conduct of the study. If, during the course of the study, the animals contract such a disease or condition, the diseased animals shall be Isolated, if necessary. These animals may be treated for disease or signs of disease provided that such treatment does not interfere with the study. The diagnosis, authorizations of treatment, description of treatment, and each date of treatment shall be documented and shall be retained.

(d) Warm-blooded animals, excluding suckling rodents, used In laboratory procedures that require manipulations and observations over an extended period of time or in studies that require the animals to be removed from and returned to their home cages for any reason (e.g., cage cleaning, treatment, etc.), shall receive appropriate identification. All information needed to specifically identify each animal within an animal-housing unit shall appear on the outside of that unit.

(e) Animals of different species shall be housed in separate rooms when necessary. Animals of the same species, but used in different studies, should not ordinarily be housed in the same room when inadvertent exposure to control or test articles or animal mixup could affect the outcome of either study. If such mixed housing is necessary, adequate differentiation by space and identification shall be made.

(f) Animal cages, racks and accessory equipment shall be cleaned and sanitized at appropriate intervals.

(g) Feed and water used for the animals shall be analyzed periodically to ensure that contaminants known to be capable of interfering with the study and reasonably expected to be present in such feed or water are not present at levels above those specified in the protocol. Documentation of such analyses shall be maintained as raw data.

(h) Bedding used in animal cages or pens shall not interfere with the purpose or conduct of the study and shall be changed as often as necessary to keep the animals dry and clean.

(i) If any pest control materials are used, the use shall be documented. Cleaning and pest control materials that interfere with the study shall not be used.

(Information collection requirements approved by the Office of Management and Budget under control number 0910-0203).

[43 FR 60013, Dec. 22, 1978, as amended at 52 FR 33780, Sept. 4, 1987; 54 FR 15924, Apr. 20, 1989; 56 FR 32088, July 15, 1991]

Subpart F - Test and Control Articles

Sec. 58.105 Test and control article characterization.

(a) The identity, strength, purity, and composition or other characteristics which will appropriately define the test or control article shall be determined for each batch and shall be documented. Methods of synthesis, fabrication, or derivation of the test and control articles shall be documented by the sponsor or the testing facility. In those cases where marketed products are used as control articles, such products will be characterized by their labeling.

(b) The stability of each test or control article shall be determined by the testing facility or by the sponsor either: (1) Before study Initiation, or (2) concomitantly according to written standard operating procedures, which provide for periodic analysis of each batch.

(c) Each storage container for a test or control article shall be labeled by name, chemical abstract number or rode number, batch number, expiration date, if any, and, where appropriate, storage conditions necessary to maintain the identity, strength, purity, and composition of the test or control article. Storage containers shall be assigned to a particular test article for the duration of the study.

(d) For studies of more than 4 weeks' duration, reserve samples from each batch of test and control articles shall be retained for the period of time provided by Sec. 58.195.

(Information collection requirements approved by the Office of Management and Budget under control number 0910-0203)

[43 FIR 60013, Dec. 22, 1978, as amended at 52 FR 33781, Sept. 4, 1987]

Sec. 58.107 Test and control article handling

Procedures shall be established for a system for the handling of the test and control articles to ensure that :

(a) There is proper storage.

(b) Distribution is made in a manner designed to preclude the possibility of contamination, deterioration, or damage.

(c) Proper identification is maintained throughout the distribution process.

(d) The receipt and distribution of each batch is documented. Such documentation shall include the date and quantity of each batch distributed or returned.

Sec. 58.113 Mixtures of articles with carriers

(a) For each test or control article that is mixed with a carrier, tests by appropriate analytical methods shall be conducted:

1. To determine the uniformity of the mixture and to determine, periodically, the concentration of the test or control article in the mixture.
2. To determine the stability of the test and control articles in the mixture as required by the conditions of the study either:
   (i) Before study initiation, or
   (ii) Concomitantly according to written standard operating procedures which provide for periodic analysis of the test and control articles in the mixture.

(b) [Reserved]

(c) Where any of the components of the test or control article carrier mixture has an expiration date, that date shall be clearly shown on the container. If more than one component has an expiration date, the earliest date shall be shown.

[43 FR 60013, Dec. 22, 1978, as amended at 45 FR 24865, Apr. 11, 1980; 52 FR 33781, Sept.4,1987]

Subpart G - Protocol for and Conduct of a Nonclinical Laboratory Study

Sec. 58.120 Protocol

(a) Each study shall have an approved written protocol that clearly indicates the objectives and all methods for the conduct of the study. The protocol shall contain, as applicable, the following information:

1. A descriptive title and statement of the purpose of the study
2. Identification of the test and control articles by name, chemical abstract number, or code number.
3. The name of the sponsor and the name and address of the testing facility at which the study is being conducted.
4. The number, body weight range, sex, source of supply, species, strain, substrain, and age of the test system.
5. The procedure for identification of the test system.

6. A description of the experimental design, including the methods for the control of bias.
7. A description and/or identification of the diet used in the study as well as solvents, emulsifiers, and/or other materials used to solubilize or suspend the test or control articles before mixing with the carrier. The description shall include specifications for acceptable levels of contaminants that are reasonably expected to be present in the dietary materials and are known to be capable of interfering with the purpose or conduct of the study if present at levels greater than established by the specifications.
8. Each dosage level, expressed In milligrams per kilogram of body weight or other appropriate units, of the test or control article to be administered and the method and frequency of administration.
9. The type and frequency of tests, analyses, and measurements to be made.
10. The records to be maintained.
11. The date of approval of the protocol by the sponsor and the dated signature of the study director.
12. A statement of the proposed statistical methods to be used.

(b) All changes In or revisions of an approved protocol and the reasons therefor shall be documented, signed by the study director, dated, and maintained with the protocol.

(Information collection requirements approved by the Office of Management and Budget under control number 0910-0203).

43 FR 60013, Dec. 22, 1978, as amended at 52 FR 33781, Sept. 4, 1987]

Sec. 58.130 Conduct of a nonclinical laboratory study

(a) The nonclinical laboratory study shall be conducted in accordance with the protocol.

(b) The test systems shall be monitored in conformity with the protocol.

(c) Specimens shall be identified by test system, study, nature, and date of collection. This Information shall be located on the specimen container or shall accompany the specimen in a manner that precludes error in the recording and storage of data.

(d) Records of gross findings for a specimen from postmortem observations should be available to a pathologist when examining that specimen histopathologically.

(e) All data generated during the conduct of a nonclinical laboratory study, except those that are generated by automated data collection systems, shall be recorded directly, promptly, and legibly in ink. All data entries shall be dated on the date of entry and signed or initialed by the person entering the data. Any change in entries shall be made so as not to obscure the original entry, shall indicate the reason for such change, and shall be dated and signed or identified at the time of the change. In automated data collection systems, the individual responsible for direct data input shall be identified at the time of data input. Any change in automated data entries shall be made so as not to obscure the original entry, shall indicate the reason for change, shall be dated, and the responsible individual shall be identified.

(Information collection requirements approved by the Office of Management and Budget under control number 0910-0203)

[43 FR 60013, Dec. 22, 1978, as amended at 52 FR 33781, Sept. 4,1987]

Subparts H - I - [Reserved]

Subpart J - Records and Reports

Sec. 58.185 Reporting of nonclinical laboratory study results

(a) A final report shall be prepared for each nonclinical laboratory study and shall include, but not necessarily be limited to, the following :

1. Name and address of the facility performing the study and the dates on which the study was initiated and completed.
2. Objectives and procedures stated in the approved protocol, including any changes in the original protocol.
3. Statistical methods employed for analyzing the data.
4. The test and control articles identified by name, chemical abstracts number or code number, strength, purity, and composition or other appropriate characteristics.

5. Stability of the test and control articles under the conditions of administration.
6. A description of the methods used.
7. A description of the test system used. Where applicable, the final report shall include the number of animals used, sex, body weight range, source of supply, species, strain and substrain, age, and procedure used for identification.
8. A description of the dosage, dosage regimen, route of administration, and duration.
9. A description of all circumstances that may have affected the quality or integrity of the data.
10. The name of the study director, the names of other scientists or professionals, and the names of all supervisory personnel, involved in the study.
11. A description of the transformations, calculations, or operations performed on the data, a summary and analysis of the data, and a statement of the conclusions drawn from the analysis.
12. The signed and dated reports of each of the individual scientists or other professionals involved in the study.
13. The locations where all specimens, raw data, and the final report are to be stored.
14. The statement prepared and signed by the quality assurance unit as described in Sec. 58.35(b)(7).

(b) The final report shall be signed and dated by the study director.

(c) Corrections or additions to a final report shall be in the form of an amendment by the study director. The amendment shall clearly identify that part of the final report that is being added to or corrected and the reasons for the correction or addition, and shall be signed and dated by the person responsible.

[43 FR 60013, Dec. 22, 1978, as amended at 52 FR 33781, Sept. 4, 1987]

Sec. 58.190 Storage and retrieval of records and data

(a) All raw data, documentation, protocols, final reports, and specimens (except those specimens obtained from mutagenicity tests and wet specimens of blood, urine, feces, and biological fluids) generated as a result of a nonclinical laboratory study shall be retained.

(b) There shall be archives for orderly storage and expedient retrieval of all raw data, documentation, protocols, specimens, and interim and final reports. Conditions of storage shall minimize deterioration of the documents or specimens in accordance with the requirements for the time period of their retention and the nature of the documents or specimens. A testing facility may contract with commercial archives to provide a repository for all material to be retained. Raw data and specimens may be retained elsewhere provided that the archives have specific reference to those other locations.

(c) An individual shall be identified as responsible for the archives.

(d) Only authorized personnel shall enter the archives.

(e) Material retained or referred to in the archives shall be indexed to permit expedient retrieval.

(Information collection requirements approved by the Office of Management and Budget under control number 0910-0203).

[43 FR 60013, Dec. 22, 1978, as amended at 52 FR 33781, Sept. 4,1987]

Sec. 58.195 Retention of records

(a) Record retention requirements set forth in this section do not supersede the record retention requirements of any other regulations in this chapter.

(b) Except as provided in paragraph (c) of this section, documentation records, raw data and specimens pertaining to a nonclinical laboratory study and required to be made by this part shall be retained in the archive(s) for whichever of the following periods is shortest :

1. A period of at least 2 years following the date on which an application for a research or marketing permit, in support of which the results of the nonclinical laboratory study were submitted, is approved by the Food and Drug Administration. This requirement does not apply to studies supporting investigational new drug applications (IND's) or applications for investigational device exemptions (IDE's), records of which shall be governed by the provisions of paragraph (b)(2) of this section.

2. A period of at least 5 years following the date on which the results of the nonclinical laboratory study are submitted to the Food and Drug Administration in support of an application for a research or marketing permit.
3. In other situations (e.g., where the nonclinical laboratory study does not result in the submission of the study in support of an application for a research or marketing permit), a period of at least 2 years following the date on which the study is completed, terminated, or discontinued.

(c) Wet specimens (except those specimens obtained from mutagenicity tests and wet specimens of blood, urine, feces, and biological fluids), samples of test or control articles, and specially prepared material, which are relatively fragile and differ markedly in stability and quality during storage, shall be retained only as loOng as the quality of the preparation affords evaluation. In no case shall retention be required for longer periods than those set forth in paragraphs (a) and (b) of this section.

(d) The master schedule sheet, copies of protocols, and records of quality assurance inspections, as required by Sec. 58.35(c) shall be maintained by the quality assurance unit as an easily accessible system of records for the period of time specified in paragraphs (a) and (b) of this section.

(e) Summaries of training and experience and job descriptions required to be maintained by Sec. 58.29(b) may be retained along with all other testing facility employment records for the length of time specified in paragraphs (a) and (b) of this section.

(f) Records and reports of the maintenance and calibration and inspection of equipment, as required by Sec. 58.63(b) and (c) shall be retained for the length of time specified in paragraph (b) of this section.

(g) Records required by this part may be retained either as original records or as true copies such as photocopies, microfilm, microfiche, or other accurate reproductions of the original records.

(h) If a facility conducting nonclinical testing goes out of business, all raw data, documentation, and other material specified in this section shall be transferred to the archives of the sponsor of the study. The Food and Drug Administration shall be notified in writing of such a transfer.

[43 FR 60013, Dec. 22, 1978, as amended at 52 FR 33781, Sept. 4, 1987; 54 FR 9039, Mar. 3,1989]

Subpart K - Disqualification of Testing Facilities

Sec. 58.200 Purpose

(a) The purposes of disqualification are : 1. To permit the exclusion from consideration of completed studies that were conducted by a testing facility which has failed to comply with the requirements of the good laboratory practice regulations until it can be adequately demonstrated that such noncompliance did not occur during, or did not affect the validity or acceptability of data generated by, a particular study; and 2. to exclude from consideration all studies completed after the date of disqualification until the facility can satisfy the Commissioner that It will conduct studies in compliance with such regulations.

(b) The determination that a nonclinical laboratory study may not be considered in support of an application for a research or marketing permit does not, however, relieve the applicant for such a permit of any obligation under any other applicable regulation to submit the results of the study to the Food and Drug Administration.

Sec. 58.202 Grounds for disqualification

The Commissioner may disqualify a testing facility upon finding all of the following :

(a) The testing facility failed to comply with one or more of the regulations set forth in this part (or any other regulations regarding such facilities in this chapter);

(b) The noncompliance adversely affected the validity of the nonclinical laboratory studies; and

(c) Other lesser regulatory actions (e.g., warnings or rejection of individual studies) have not been or will probably not be adequate to achieve compliance with the good laboratory practice regulations.

Sec. 58.204 Notice of and opportunity or hearing on proposed disqualification

(a) Whenever the Commissioner has information indicating that grounds exist under Sec. 58.202 which in his opinion justify disqualification of a testing facility, he may issue to the testing facility a written notice proposing that the facility be disqualified.

(b) A hearing on the disqualification shall be conducted in accordance with the requirements for a regulatory hearing set forth in part 16 of this chapter.

Sec. 58.206 Final order on disqualification

(a) If the Commissioner, after the regulatory hearing, or after the time for requesting a hearing expires without a request being made, upon an evaluation of the administrative record of the disqualification proceeding, makes the findings required In Sec. 58.202, he shall issue a final order disqualifying the facility. Such order shall include a statement of the basis for that determination. Upon issuing a final order, the Commissioner shall notify (with a copy of the order) the testing facility of the action.

(b) If the Commissioner, after a regulatory hearing or after the time for requesting a hearing expires without a request being made, upon an evaluation of the administrative record of the disqualification proceeding, does not make the findings required in Sec. 58.202, he shall Issue a final order terminating the disqualification proceeding. Such order shall include a statement of the basis for that determination. Upon issuing a final order the Commissioner shall notify the testing facility and provide a copy of the order.

Sec. 58.210 Actions upon disqualification

(a) Once a testing facility has been disqualified, each application for a research or marketing permit, whether approved or not, containing or relying upon any nonclinical laboratory study conducted by the disqualified testing facility may be examined to determine whether such study was or would be essential to a decision. If it is determined that a study was or would be essential, the Food and Drug Administration shall also determine whether the study is acceptable, notwithstanding the disqualification of the facility. Any study done by a testing facility before or after disqualification may be presumed to be unacceptable, and the person relying on the study may be required to establish that the study was not affected by the circumstances that led to the disqualification, e.g., by submitting validating information. If the study is then determined to be unacceptable, such data such be eliminated from consideration in support of the application; and such elimination may serve as new Information justifying the termination or withdrawal of approval of the application.

(b) No nonclinical laboratory study begun by a testing facility after the date of the facility's disqualification shall be considered in support of any application for a research or marketing permit, unless the facility has been reinstated under Sec. 58.219. The determination that a study may not be considered in support of an application for a research or marketing permit does not, however, relieve the applicant for such a permit of any obligation under any other applicable regulation to submit the results of the study to the Food and Drug Administration.

[43 FR 60013, Dec. 22, 1978, as amended at 59 FR 13200, Mar. 21, 1994]

Sec. 58.213 Public disclosure of information regarding disqualification

(a) Upon issuance of a final order disqualifying a testing facility under Sec. 58.206(a), the Commissioner may notify all or any interested persons. Such notice may be given at the discretion of the Commissioner whenever he believes that such disclosure would further the public interest or would promote compliance with the good laboratory practice regulations set forth in this part. Such notice, if given, shall include a copy of the final order issued under Sec. 58.206(a) and shall state that the disqualification constitutes a determination by the Food and Drug Administration that nonclinical laboratory studies performed by the facility will not be considered by the Food and Drug Administration in support of any application for a research or marketing permit. If such notice is sent to another Federal Government agency, the Food and Drug Administration will recommend that the agency also consider whether or not it should accept nonclinical laboratory studies performed by the testing facility. If such notice is sent to any other person, it shallstate that it is given because of the relationship between the testing facility and the person being notified and that the Food and Drug Administration is not advising or recommending that any action be taken by the person notified.

(b) A determination that a testing facility has been disqualified and the administrative record regarding such determination are disclosable to the public under part 20 of this chapter.

Sec. 58.215 Alternative or additional actions to disqualification.

(a) Disqualification of a testing facility under this subpart is independent of, and neither in lieu of nor a precondition to, other proceedings or actions authorized by the act. The Food and Drug Administration may, at any time, institute against a testing facility and/ or against the sponsor of a nonclinical laboratory study that has been submitted to the Food and Drug Administration any appropriate judicial proceedings (civil or criminal) and any other appropriate regulatory action, in addition to or in lieu of, and prior to, simultaneously with, or subsequent to, disqualification. The Food and Drug Administration may also refer the matter to another Federal, State, or local government law enforcement or regulatory agency for such action as that agency deems appropriate.

(b) The Food and Drug Administration may refuse to consider any particular nonclinical laboratory study in support of an application for a research or marketing permit, if it finds that the study was not conducted in accordance with the good laboratory practice regulations set forth in this part, without disqualifying the testing facility that conducted the study or undertaking other regulatory action.

Sec. 58.217 Suspension or termination of a testing facility by a sponsor

Termination of a testing facility by a sponsor is independent of, and neither in lieu of nor a precondition to, proceedings or actions authorized by this subpart. If a sponsor terminates or suspends a testing facility from further participation in a nonclinical laboratory study that is being conducted as part of any application for a research or marketing permit that has been submitted to any Center of the Food and Drug Administration (whether approved or not), it shall notify that Center in writing within 15 working days of the action; the notice shall include a statement of the reasons for such action. Suspension or termination of a testing facility by a sponsor does not relieve it of any obligation under any other applicable regulation to submit the results of the study to the Food and Drug Administration.

[43 FR FR 60013, Dec. 22, 1978, as amended at 50 FR 8995, Mar. 6, 1985]

58.219 Reinstatement of a disqualified testing facility

A testing facility that has been disqualified may be reinstated as an acceptable source of nonclinical laboratory studies to be submitted to the Food and Drug Administration if the Commissioner determines, upon an evaluation of the submission of the testing facility, that the facility can adequately assure that it will conduct future nonclinical laboratory studies in compliance with the good laboratory practice regulations set forth in this part and, if any studies are currently being conducted, that the quality and integrity of such studies have not been seriously compromised. A disqualified testing facility that wishes to be so reinstated shall present in writing to the Commissioner reasons why it believes it should be reinstated and a detailed description of the corrective actions it has taken or intends to take to assure that the acts or omissions which led to its disqualification will not recur. The Commissioner may condition reinstatement upon the testing facility being found in compliance with the good laboratory practice regulations upon an inspection. If a testing facility is reinstated, the Commissioner shall so notify the testing facility and all organizations and persons who were notified, under Sec. 58.213 of the disqualification of the testing facility. A determination that a testing facility has been reinstated is disclosable to the public under part 20 of this chapter.

Go to :

Other Federal Animal Care Legislation and Policies
Top of Document

The Animal Welfare Information Center
U.S. Department of Agriculture
Agricultural Research Service
National Agricultural Library
10301 Baltimore Ave.
Beltsville, MD 20705-2351

Phone : (301) 504-6212
FAX : (301) 504-7125
E-mail : awic@nal.usda.gov

June 1998

This page's URL is http://www.nal.usda.gov/awic/legislat/21cfr97.htm

Appendix-III

Guidance for Industry
Q7A Good Manufacturing Practice Guidance for Active Pharmaceutical Ingredients

U.S. Department of Health and Human Services

Food and Drug Administration
Center for Drug Evaluation and Research (CDER)
Center for Biologics Evaluation and Research (CBER)
August 2001
ICH

Additional copies are available from :

Office of Training and Communications
Division of Communications Management
Drug Information Branch, HFD-210
5600 Fishers Lane
Rockville, MD 20857
(Tel) 301-827-4573
(Internet) http://www.fda.gov/cder/guidance/index.htm

or

Office of Communication, Training and
Manufacturers Assistance, HFM-40
Center for Biologics Evaluation and Research
Food and Drug Administration
1401 Rockville Pike, Rockville, MD 20852-1448
Internet: http://www.fda.gov/cber/guidelines.htm
Fax: 1-888-CBERFAX or 301-827-3844
Mail: the Voice Information System at 800-835-4709 or
301-827-1800

August 2001

ICH

Table Of Contents

IV. BUILDINGS AND FACILITIES (4)

A. Design and Construction (4.1)
B. Utilities (4.2)
C. Water (4.3)
D. Containment (4.4)
E. Lighting (4.5)
F. Sewage and Refuse (4.6)
G. Sanitation and Maintenance (4.7)

V. PROCESS EQUIPMENT (5)

A. Design and Construction (5.1)
B. Equipment Maintenance and Cleaning (5.2)
C. Calibration (5.3)
D. Computerized Systems (5.4)

VI. DOCUMENTATION AND RECORDS (6)

A. Documentation System and Specifications (6.1)
B. Equipment Cleaning and Use Record (6.2)
C. Records of Raw Materials, Intermediates, API Labeling and Packaging Materials (6.3)
D. Master Production Instructions (Master Production and Control Records) (6.4)
E. Batch Production Records (Batch Production and Control Records) (6.5)
F. Laboratory Control Records (6.6)
G. Batch Production Record Review (6.7)

VII MATERIALS MANAGEMENT (7)

A. General Controls (7.1)
B. Receipt and Quarantine (7.2)
C. Sampling and Testing of Incoming Production Materials (7.3)
D. Storage (7.4)
E. Re-evaluation (7.5)

VIII PRODUCTION AND IN-PROCESS CONTROLS (8)

A. Production Operations (8.1)

B. Time Limits (8.2)

C. In-process Sampling and Controls (8.3)

D. Blending Batches of Intermediates or APIs (8.4)

E. Contamination Control (8.5)

IX PACKAGING AND IDENTIFICATION LABELING OF APIs AND INTERMEDIATES (9)

A. General (9.1)

B. Packaging Materials (9.2)

C. Label Issuance and Control (9.3)

D. Packaging and Labeling Operations (9.4)

X. STORAGE AND DISTRIBUTION (10)

A. Warehousing Procedures (10.1)

B. Distribution Procedures (10.2)

XI. LABORATORY CONTROLS (11)

A. General Controls (11.1)

B. Testing of Intermediates and APIs (11.2)

C. Validation of Analytical Procedures - See Section 12. (11.3)

D. Certificates of Analysis (11.4)

E. Stability Monitoring of APIs (11.5)

F. Expiry and Retest Dating (11.6)

G. Reserve/Retention Samples (11.7)

XII. VALIDATION (12)

A. Validation Policy (12.1)

B. Validation Documentation (12.2)

C. Qualification (12.3)

D. Approaches to Process Validation (12.4)

E. Process Validation Program (12.5)

F. Periodic Review of Validated Systems (12.6)

G. Cleaning Validation (12.7)

H. Validation of Analytical Methods (12.8)

XIII. CHANGE CONTROL (13)

XIV. REJECTION AND RE-USE OF MATERIALS (14)

A. Rejection (14.1)

B. Reprocessing (14.2)

C. Reworking (14.3)

D. Recovery of Materials and Solvents (14.4)

E. Returns (14.5)

XV. COMPLAINTS AND RECALLS (15)

XVI. CONTRACT MANUFACTURERS (INCLUDING LABORATORIES) (16)

XVII. AGENTS, BROKERS, TRADERS, DISTRIBUTORS, REPACKERS, AND RELABELLERS (17)

A. Applicability (17.1)

B. Traceability of Distributed APIs and Intermediates (17.2)

C. Quality Management (17.3)

D. Repackaging, Relabeling, and Holding of APIs and Intermediates (17.4)

E. Stability (17.5)

F. Transfer of Information (17.6)

G. Handling of Complaints and Recalls (17.7)

H. Handling of Returns (17.8)

XVIII. SPECIFIC GUIDANCE FOR APIs MANUFACTURED BY CELL CULTURE/FERMENTATION (18)

A. General (18.1)

B. Cell Bank Maintenance and Record Keeping (18.2)

C. Cell Culture/Fermentation (18.3)

D. Harvesting, Isolation and Purification (18.4)

E. Viral Removal/Inactivation steps (18.5)

XIX APIs FOR USE IN CLINICAL TRIALS (19)

A. General (19.1)

B. Quality (19.2)

C. Equipment and Facilities (19.3)

D. Control of Raw Materials (19.4)

E. Production (19.5)

F. Validation (19.6)

G. Changes (19.7)

H. Laboratory Controls (19.8)

I. Documentation (19.9)

XX Glossary

Q7A Good Manufacturing Practice Guidance for Active Pharmaceutical Ingredients

This guidance represents the Food and Drug Administration's (FDA's) current thinking on this topic. It does not create or confer any rights for or on any person and does not operate to bind FDA or the public. An alternative approach may be used if such approach satisfies the requirements of the applicable statutes and regulations.

I. Introduction (1)

A. Objective (1.1)

This document is intended to provide guidance regarding good manufacturing practice (GMP) for the manufacturing of active pharmaceutical ingredients (APIs) under an appropriate system for managing quality. It is also intended to help ensure that APIs meet the quality and purity characteristics that they purport, or are represented, to possess.

In this guidance, the term *manufacturing* is defined to include all operations of receipt of materials, production, packaging, repackaging, labeling, relabeling, quality control, release, storage and distribution of APIs and the related controls. In this guidance, the term *should* identifies recommendations that, when followed, will ensure compliance with CGMPs. An alternative approach may be used if such approach satisfies the requirements of the applicable statutes. For the purposes of this guidance, the terms *current good manufacturing practices* and *good manufacturing practices* are equivalent.

The guidance as a whole does not cover safety aspects for the personnel engaged in manufacturing, nor aspects related to protecting the environment. These controls are inherent responsibilities of the manufacturer and are governed by national laws.

This guidance is not intended to define registration and/or filing requirements or modify pharmacopoeial requirements. This guidance does not affect the ability of the responsible regulatory agency to establish specific registration/filing requirements regarding APIs within the context of marketing/manufacturing authorizations or drug applications. All commitments in registration/filing documents should be met.

B. Regulatory Applicability (1.2)

Within the world community, materials may vary as to their legal classification as an API. When a material is classified as an API in the region or country in which it is manufactured or used in a drug product, it should be manufactured according to this guidance.

C. Scope (1.3)

This guidance applies to the manufacture of APIs for use in human drug (medicinal) products. It applies to the manufacture of sterile APIs only up to the point immediately prior to the APIs being rendered sterile. The sterilization and aseptic processing of sterile APIs are not covered by this guidance, but should be performed in accordance with GMP guidances for drug (medicinal) products as defined by local authorities.

This guidance covers APIs that are manufactured by chemical synthesis, extraction, cell culture/fermentation, recovery from natural sources, or any combination of these processes. Specific guidance for APIs manufactured by cell culture/fermentation is described in Section XVIII (18).

This guidance excludes all vaccines, whole cells, whole blood and plasma, blood and plasma derivatives (plasma fractionation), and gene therapy APIs. However, it does include APIs that are produced using blood or plasma as raw materials. Note that cell substrates (mammalian, plant, insect or microbial cells, tissue or animal sources including transgenic animals) and early process steps may be subject to GMP but are not covered by this guidance. In addition, the guidance does not apply to medical gases, bulk-packaged drug (medicinal) products (e.g., tablets or capsules in bulk containers), or radiopharmaceuticals.

Section XIX (19) contains guidance that only applies to the manufacture of APIs used in the production of drug (medicinal) products specifically for clinical trials (investigational medicinal products).

An *API starting material* is a raw material, an intermediate, or an API that is used in the production of an API and that is incorporated as a significant structural fragment into the structure of the API. An API starting material can be an article of commerce, a material purchased from one or more suppliers under contract or commercial agreement, or produced in-house. API starting materials normally have defined chemical properties and structure.

The company should designate and document the rationale for the point at which production of the API begins. For synthetic processes, this is known as the point at which API starting materials are entered into the process. For other processes (e.g., fermentation, extraction, purification), this rationale should be established on a case-by-case basis. Table 1 gives guidance on the point at which the API starting material is normally introduced into the process.

From this point on, appropriate GMP as defined in this guidance should be applied to these intermediate and/or API manufacturing steps. This would include the validation of critical process steps determined to impact the quality of the API. However, it should be noted that the fact that a company chooses to validate a process step does not necessarily define that step as critical.

The guidance in this document would normally be applied to the steps shown in gray in Table 1. However, all steps shown may not need to be completed. The stringency of GMP in API manufacturing should increase as the process proceeds from early API steps to final steps, purification, and packaging. Physical processing of APIs, such as granulation, coating or physical manipulation of particle size (e.g., milling, micronizing) should be conducted according to this guidance.

This GMP guidance does not apply to steps prior to the introduction of the defined API starting material.

Table 1 Application of this Guidance to API Manufacturing

Type of Manufacturing	**Application of this guidance to steps (shown in gray) used in this type of manufacturing**				
Chemical Manufacturing	Production of the API starting material	Introduction of the API starting material into process	Production of Intermediate(s)	Isolation and purification	Physical processing, and packaging
API derived from animal sources	Collection of organ, fluid, or tissue	Cutting, mixing, and/or initial processing	Introduction of the API starting process material into process	Isolation and purification	Physical processing, and packaging
API extracted from plant sources	Collection of plant	Cutting and initial extraction(s)	Introduction of the API starting material into process	Isolation and purification	Physical processing, and packaging
Herbal extracts used as API	Collection of plants extraction	Cutting and initial		Further extraction	Physical processing, and packaging
API consisting of comminuted or powdered herbs	Collection of plants and/or cultivation and harvesting	Cutting/ comminuting			Physical processing, and packaging
Biotechnology : fermentation/	Establishment of cell culture master cell bank and working cell bank	Maintenance of working cell bank	Cell culture and/or fermentation	Isolation and purification	Physical processing, and packaging
"Classical" Fermentation to produce an API	Establish-ment of cell bank	Maintenance of the cell bank	Introduction of the cells into fermentation	Isolation and purification	Physical processing, and packaging

Increasing GMP Requirements

II. QUALITY MANAGEMENT (2)

A. Principles (2.1)

Quality should be the responsibility of all persons involved in manufacturing.

Each manufacturer should establish, document, and implement an effective system for managing quality that involves the active participation of management and appropriate manufacturing personnel.

The system for managing quality should encompass the organizational structure, procedures, processes and resources, as well as activities to ensure confidence that the API will meet its intended specifications for quality and purity. All quality-related activities should be defined and documented.

There should be a quality unit(s) that is independent of production and that fulfills both quality assurance *(QA)* and quality control *(QC)* responsibilities. The quality unit can be in the form of separate QA and QC units or a single individual or group, depending upon the size and structure of the organization.

The persons authorized to release intermediates and APIs should be specified.

All quality-related activities should be recorded at the time they are performed.

Any deviation from established procedures should be documented and explained. Critical deviations should be investigated, and the investigation and its conclusions should be documented.

No materials should be released or used before the satisfactory completion of evaluation by the quality unit(s) unless there are appropriate systems in place to allow for such use (e.g., release under quarantine as described in Section X (10) or the use of raw materials or intermediates pending completion of evaluation).

Procedures should exist for notifying responsible management in a timely manner of regulatory inspections, serious GMP deficiencies, product defects and related actions (e.g., quality-related complaints, recalls, and regulatory actions).

B. Responsibilities of the Quality Unit(s) (2.2)

The quality unit(s) should be involved in all quality-related matters.

The quality unit(s) should review and approve all appropriate quality-related documents.

The main responsibilities of the independent quality unit(s) should not be delegated. These responsibilities should be described in writing and should include, but not necessarily be limited to :

1. Releasing or rejecting all APIs. Releasing or rejecting intermediates for use outside the control of the manufacturing company.
2. Establishing a system to release or reject raw materials, intermediates, packaging, and labeling materials.
3. Reviewing completed batch production and laboratory control records of critical process steps before release of the API for distribution.
4. Making sure that critical deviations are investigated and resolved.
5. Approving all specifications and master production instructions.
6. Approving all procedures affecting the quality of intermediates or APIs.
7. Making sure that internal audits (self-inspections) are performed.
8. Approving intermediate and API contract manufacturers.
9. Approving changes that potentially affect intermediate or API quality.
10. Reviewing and approving validation protocols and reports.
11. Making sure that quality-related complaints are investigated and resolved.
12. Making sure that effective systems are used for maintaining and calibrating critical equipment.
13. Making sure that materials are appropriately tested and the results are reported.
14. Making sure that there is stability data to support retest or expiry dates and storage conditions on APIs and/or intermediates, where appropriate
15. Performing product quality reviews (as defined in Section 2.5)

C. Responsibility for Production Activities (2.3)

The responsibility for production activities should be described in writing and should include, but not necessarily be limited to :

1. Preparing, reviewing, approving, and distributing the instructions for the production of intermediates or APIs according to written procedures.
2. Producing APIs and, when appropriate, intermediates according to pre-approved instructions.
3. Reviewing all production batch records and ensuring that these are completed and signed.
4. Making sure that all production deviations are reported and evaluated and that critical deviations are investigated and the conclusions are recorded.
5. Making sure that production facilities are clean and, when appropriate, disinfected.
6. Making sure that the necessary calibrations are performed and records kept.
7. Making sure that the premises and equipment are maintained and records kept.
8. Making sure that validation protocols and reports are reviewed and approved.
9. Evaluating proposed changes in product, process or equipment.
10. Making sure that new and, when appropriate, modified facilities and equipment are qualified.

D. Internal Audits (Self Inspection) (2.4)

To verify compliance with the principles of GMP for APIs, regular internal audits should be performed in accordance with an approved schedule.

Audit findings and corrective actions should be documented and brought to the attention of responsible management of the firm. Agreed corrective actions should be completed in a timely and effective manner.

E. Product Quality Review (2.5)

Regular quality-reviews of APIs should be conducted with the objective of verifying the consistency of the process. Such reviews should normally be conducted and documented annually and should include at least :

- A review of critical in-process control and critical API test results
- A review of all batches that failed to meet established specification(s)

- A review of all critical deviations or nonconformances and related investigations
- A review of any changes carried out to the processes or analytical methods;
- A review of results of the stability monitoring program
- A review of all quality-related returns, complaints and recalls
- A review of adequacy of corrective actions

The results of this review should be evaluated and an assessment made of whether corrective action or any revalidation should be undertaken. Reasons for such corrective action should be documented. Agreed corrective actions should be completed in a timely and effective manner.

III. PERSONNEL (3)

A. Personnel Qualifications (3.1)

There should be an adequate number of personnel qualified by appropriate education, training, and/or experience to perform and supervise the manufacture of intermediates and APIs.

The responsibilities of all personnel engaged in the manufacture of intermediates and APIs should be specified in writing.

Training should be regularly conducted by qualified individuals and should cover, at a minimum, the particular operations that the employee performs and GMP as it relates to the employee's functions. Records of training should be maintained. Training should be periodically assessed.

B. Personnel Hygiene (3.2)

Personnel should practice good sanitation and health habits.

Personnel should wear clean clothing suitable for the manufacturing activity with which they are involved and this clothing should be changed, when appropriate. Additional protective apparel, such as head, face, hand, and arm coverings, should be worn, when necessary, to protect intermediates and APIs from contamination.

Personnel should avoid direct contact with intermediates or APIs.

Smoking, eating, drinking, chewing and the storage of food should be restricted to certain designated areas separate from the manufacturing areas.

Personnel suffering from an infectious disease or having open lesions on the exposed surface of the body should not engage in activities that could result in compromising the quality of APIs. Any person shown at any time (either by medical examination or supervisory observation) to have an apparent illness or open lesions should be excluded from activities where the health condition could adversely affect the quality of the APIs until the condition is corrected or qualified medical personnel determine that the person's inclusion would not jeopardize the safety or quality of the APIs.

C. Consultants (3.3)

Consultants advising on the manufacture and control of intermediates or APIs should have sufficient education, training, and experience, or any combination thereof, to advise on the subject for which they are retained.

Records should be maintained stating the name, address, qualifications, and type of service provided by these consultants.

IV. BUILDINGS AND FACILITIES (4)

A. Design and Construction (4.1)

Buildings and facilities used in the manufacture of intermediates and APIs should be located, designed, and constructed to facilitate cleaning, maintenance, and operations as appropriate to the type and stage of manufacture. Facilities should also be designed to minimize potential contamination. Where microbiological specifications have been established for the intermediate or API, facilities should also be designed to limit exposure to objectionable microbiological contaminants, as appropriate.

Buildings and facilities should have adequate space for the orderly placement of equipment and materials to prevent mix-ups and contamination.

Where the equipment itself (e.g., closed or contained systems) provides adequate protection of the material, such equipment can be located outdoors.

The flow of materials and personnel through the building or facilities should be designed to prevent mix-ups or contamination.

There should be defined areas or other control systems for the following activities :

- Receipt, identification, sampling, and quarantine of incoming materials, pending release or rejection.
- Quarantine before release or rejection of intermediates and APIs.
- Sampling of intermediates and APIs.

- Holding rejected materials before further disposition (e.g., return, reprocessing or destruction).
- Storage of released materials.
- Production operations.
- Packaging and labeling operations.
- Laboratory operations

Adequate and clean washing and toilet facilities should be provided for personnel. These facilities should be equipped with hot and cold water, as appropriate, soap or detergent, air dryers, or single service towels. The washing and toilet facilities should be separate from, but easily accessible to, manufacturing areas. Adequate facilities for showering and/or changing clothes should be provided, when appropriate.

Laboratory areas/operations should normally be separated from production areas. Some laboratory areas, in particular those used for in-process controls, can be located in production areas, provided the operations of the production process do not adversely affect the accuracy of the laboratory measurements, and the laboratory and its operations do not adversely affect the production process, intermediate, or API.

B. Utilities (4.2)

All utilities that could affect product quality (e.g., steam, gas, compressed air, heating, ventilation, and air conditioning) should be qualified and appropriately monitored and action should be taken when limits are exceeded. Drawings for these utility systems should be available.

Adequate ventilation, air filtration and exhaust systems should be provided, where appropriate. These systems should be designed and constructed to minimize risks of contamination and cross-contamination and should include equipment for control of air pressure, microorganisms (if appropriate), dust, humidity, and temperature, as appropriate to the stage of manufacture. Particular attention should be given to areas where APIs are exposed to the environment.

If air is recirculated to production areas, appropriate measures should be taken to control risks of contamination and cross-contamination.

Permanently installed pipework should be appropriately identified. This can be accomplished by identifying individual lines, documentation, computer control systems, or alternative means. Pipework should be located to avoid risks of contamination of the intermediate or API.

Drains should be of adequate size and should be provided with an air break or a suitable device to prevent back-siphonage, when appropriate.

C. Water (4.3)

Water used in the manufacture of APIs should be demonstrated to be suitable for its intended use.

Unless otherwise justified, process water should, at a minimum, meet World Health Organization (WHO) guidelines for drinking (potable) water quality.

If drinking (potable) water is insufficient to ensure API quality and tighter chemical and/or microbiological water quality specifications are called for, appropriate specifications for physical/chemical attributes, total microbial counts, objectionable organisms, and/or endotoxins should be established.

Where water used in the process is treated by the manufacturer to achieve a defined quality, the treatment process should be validated and monitored with appropriate action limits.

Where the manufacturer of a nonsterile API either intends or claims that it is suitable for use in further processing to produce a sterile drug (medicinal) product, water used in the final isolation and purification steps should be monitored and controlled for total microbial counts, objectionable organisms, and endotoxins.

D. Containment (4.4)

Dedicated production areas, which can include facilities, air handling equipment and/or process equipment, should be employed in the production of highly sensitizing materials, such as penicillins or cephalosporins.

The use of dedicated production areas should also be considered when material of an infectious nature or high pharmacological activity or toxicity is involved (e.g., certain steroids or cytotoxic anti-cancer agents) unless validated inactivation and/or cleaning procedures are established and maintained.

Appropriate measures should be established and implemented to prevent cross-contamination from personnel and materials moving from one dedicated area to another.

Any production activities (including weighing, milling, or packaging) of highly toxic nonpharmaceutical materials, such as herbicides and pesticides, should not be conducted using the buildings and/or equipment being used for the production of APIs. Handling and storage of these highly toxic nonpharmaceutical materials should be separate from APIs.

E. Lighting (4.5)

Adequate lighting should be provided in all areas to facilitate cleaning, maintenance, and proper operations.

F. Sewage and Refuse (4.6)

Sewage, refuse, and other waste (e.g., solids, liquids, or gaseous by-products from manufacturing) in and from buildings and the immediate surrounding area should be disposed of in a safe, timely, and sanitary manner. Containers and/or pipes for waste material should be clearly identified.

G. Sanitation and Maintenance (4.7)

Buildings used in the manufacture of intermediates and APIs should be properly maintained and repaired and kept in a clean condition.

Written procedures should be established assigning responsibility for sanitation and describing the cleaning schedules, methods, equipment, and materials to be used in cleaning buildings and facilities.

When necessary, written procedures should also be established for the use of suitable rodenticides, insecticides, fungicides, fumigating agents, and cleaning and sanitizing agents to prevent the contamination of equipment, raw materials, packaging/labeling materials, intermediates, and APIs.

V. PROCESS EQUIPMENT (5)

A. Design and Construction (5.1)

Equipment used in the manufacture of intermediates and APIs should be of appropriate design and adequate size, and suitably located for its intended use, cleaning, sanitation (where appropriate), and maintenance.

Equipment should be constructed so that surfaces that contact raw materials, intermediates, or APIs do not alter the quality of the intermediates and APIs beyond the official or other established specifications.

Production equipment should only be used within its qualified operating range.

Major equipment (e.g., reactors, storage containers) and permanently installed processing lines used during the production of an intermediate or API should be appropriately identified.

Any substances associated with the operation of equipment, such as lubricants, heating fluids or coolants, should not contact intermediates or APIs so as to alter the quality of APIs or intermediates beyond the official or other established specifications. Any deviations from this practice should be evaluated to ensure that there are no detrimental effects on the material's fitness for use. Wherever possible, food grade lubricants and oils should be used.

Closed or contained equipment should be used whenever appropriate. Where open equipment is used, or equipment is opened, appropriate precautions should be taken to minimize the risk of contamination.

A set of current drawings should be maintained for equipment and critical installations (e.g., instrumentation and utility systems).

B. Equipment Maintenance and Cleaning (5.2)

Schedules and procedures (including assignment of responsibility) should be established for the preventative maintenance of equipment.

Written procedures should be established for cleaning equipment and its subsequent release for use in the manufacture of intermediates and APIs. Cleaning procedures should contain sufficient details to enable operators to clean each type of equipment in a reproducible and effective manner. These procedures should include :

- Assignment of responsibility for cleaning of equipment.
- Cleaning schedules, including, where appropriate, sanitizing schedules.
- A complete description of the methods and materials, including dilution of cleaning agents used to clean equipment.
- When appropriate, instructions for disassembling and reassembling each article of equipment to ensure proper cleaning.
- Instructions for the removal or obliteration of previous batch identification.
- Instructions for the protection of clean equipment from contamination prior to use.
- Inspection of equipment for cleanliness immediately before use, if practical.
- Establishing the maximum time that may elapse between the completion of processing and equipment cleaning, when appropriate.

- Equipment and utensils should be cleaned, stored, and, where appropriate, sanitized or sterilized to prevent contamination or carry-over of a material that would alter the quality of the intermediate or API beyond the official or other established specifications.

Where equipment is assigned to continuous production or campaign production of successive batches of the same intermediate or API, equipment should be cleaned at appropriate intervals to prevent build-up and carry-over of contaminants (e.g., degradants or objectionable levels of microorganisms).

Nondedicated equipment should be cleaned between production of different materials to prevent cross-contamination.

Acceptance criteria for residues and the choice of cleaning procedures and cleaning agents should be defined and justified.

Equipment should be identified as to its contents and its cleanliness status by appropriate means.

C. Calibration (5.3)

Control, weighing, measuring, monitoring, and testing equipment critical for ensuring the quality of intermediates or APIs should be calibrated according to written procedures and an established schedule.

Equipment calibrations should be performed using standards traceable to certified standards, if they exist.

Records of these calibrations should be maintained.

The current calibration status of critical equipment should be known and verifiable.

Instruments that do not meet calibration criteria should not be used.

Deviations from approved standards of calibration on critical instruments should be investigated to determine if these could have had an effect on the quality of the intermediate(s) or API(s) manufactured using this equipment since the last successful calibration.

D. Computerized Systems (5.4)

GMP-related computerized systems should be validated. The depth and scope of validation depends on the diversity, complexity, and criticality of the computerized application.

Appropriate installation and operational qualifications should demonstrate the suitability of computer hardware and software to perform assigned tasks.

Commercially available software that has been qualified does not require the same level of testing. If an existing system was not validated at time of installation, a retrospective validation could be conducted if appropriate documentation is available.

Computerized systems should have sufficient controls to prevent unauthorized access or changes to data. There should be controls to prevent omissions in data (e.g., system turned off and data not captured). There should be a record of any data change made, the previous entry, who made the change, and when the change was made.

Written procedures should be available for the operation and maintenance of computerized systems.

Where critical data are being entered manually, there should be an additional check on the accuracy of the entry. This can be done by a second operator or by the system itself.

Incidents related to computerized systems that could affect the quality of intermediates or APIs or the reliability of records or test results should be recorded and investigated.

Changes to computerized systems should be made according to a change procedure and should be formally authorized, documented, and tested. Records should be kept of all changes, including modifications and enhancements made to the hardware, software, and any other critical component of the system. These records should demonstrate that the system is maintained in a validated state.

If system breakdowns or failures would result in the permanent loss of records, a back-up system should be provided. A means of ensuring data protection should be established for all computerized systems.

Data can be recorded by a second means in addition to the computer system.

VI. DOCUMENTATION AND RECORDS (6)

A. Documentation System and Specifications (6.1)

All documents related to the manufacture of intermediates or APIs should be prepared, reviewed, approved, and distributed according to written procedures. Such documents can be in paper or electronic form.

The issuance, revision, superseding, and withdrawal of all documents should be controlled by maintaining revision histories.

A procedure should be established for retaining all appropriate documents (e.g., development history reports, scale-up reports, technical transfer reports, process validation reports, training records, production records, control records, and distribution records). The retention periods for these documents should be specified.

All production, control, and distribution records should be retained for at least 1 year after the expiry date of the batch. For APIs with retest dates, records should be retained for at least 3 years after the batch is completely distributed.

When entries are made in records, these should be made indelibly in spaces provided for such entries, directly after performing the activities, and should identify the person making the entry. Corrections to entries should be dated and signed and leave the original entry still legible.

During the retention period, originals or copies of records should be readily available at the establishment where the activities described in such records occurred. Records that can be promptly retrieved from another location by electronic or other means are acceptable.

Specifications, instructions, procedures, and records can be retained either as originals or as true copies such as photocopies, microfilm, microfiche, or other accurate reproductions of the original records. Where reduction techniques such as microfilming or electronic records are used, suitable retrieval equipment and a means to produce a hard copy should be readily available.

Specifications should be established and documented for raw materials, intermediates where necessary, APIs, and labeling and packaging materials. In addition, specifications may be appropriate for certain other materials, such as process aids, gaskets, or other materials used during the production of intermediates or APIs that could critically affect quality. Acceptance criteria should be established and documented for in-process controls.

If electronic signatures are used on documents, they should be authenticated and secure.

B. Equipment Cleaning and Use Record (6.2)

Records of major equipment use, cleaning, sanitation, and/or sterilization and maintenance should show the date, time (if appropriate), product, and batch number of each batch processed in the equipment and the person who performed the cleaning and maintenance.

If equipment is dedicated to manufacturing one intermediate or API, individual equipment records are not necessary if batches of the intermediate or API follow in traceable sequence. In cases where dedicated equipment is employed, the records of cleaning, maintenance, and use can be part of the batch record or maintained separately.

C. Records of Raw Materials, Intermediates, API Labeling and Packaging Materials (6.3)

Records should be maintained including :

- The name of the manufacturer, identity, and quantity of each shipment of each batch of raw materials, intermediates, or labeling and packaging materials for API's; the name of the supplier; the supplier's control number(s), if known, or other identification number; the number allocated on receipt; and the date of receipt.
- The results of any test or examination performed and the conclusions derived from this.
- Records tracing the use of materials
- Documentation of the examination and review of API labeling and packaging materials for conformity with established specifications
- The final decision regarding rejected raw materials, intermediates, or API labeling and packaging materials

  Master (approved) labels should be maintained for comparison to issued labels.

D. Master Production Instructions (Master Production and Control Records) (6.4)

To ensure uniformity from batch to batch, master production instructions for each intermediate and API should be prepared, dated, and signed by one person and independently checked, dated, and signed by a person in the quality unit(s).

Master production instructions should include :

- The name of the intermediate or API being manufactured and an identifying document reference code, if applicable
- A complete list of raw materials and intermediates designated by names or codes sufficiently specific to identify any special quality characteristics.

- An accurate statement of the quantity or ratio of each raw material or intermediate to be used, including the unit of measure. Where the quantity is not fixed, the calculation for each batch size or rate of production should be included. Variations to quantities should be included where they are justified.
- The production location and major production equipment to be used
- Detailed production instructions, including the :
  - sequences to be followed.
  - ranges of process parameters to be used.
  - sampling instructions and in-process controls with their acceptance criteria, where appropriate.
  - time limits for completion of individual processing steps and/or the total process, where appropriate.
  - expected yield ranges at appropriate phases of processing or time.
- Where appropriate, special notations and precautions to be followed, or cross-references to these.
- The instructions for storage of the intermediate or API to ensure its suitability for use, including the labelling and packaging materials and special storage conditions with time limits, where appropriate.

E. Batch Production Records (Batch Production and Control Records) (6.5)

Batch production records should be prepared for each intermediate and API and should include complete information relating to the production and control of each batch. The batch production record should be checked before issuance to ensure that it is the correct version and a legible accurate reproduction of the appropriate master production instruction. If the batch production record is produced from a separate part of the master document, that document should include a reference to the current master production instruction being used.

These records should be numbered with a unique batch or identification number, dated and signed when issued. In continuous production, the product code together with the date and time can serve as the unique identifier until the final number is allocated.

Documentation of completion of each significant step in the batch production records (batch production and control records) should include :

- Dates and, when appropriate, times.
- Identity of major equipment (e.g., reactors, driers, mills, etc.) used.
- Specific identification of each batch, including weights, measures, and batch numbers of raw materials, intermediates, or any reprocessed materials used during manufacturing.
- Actual results recorded for critical process parameters.
- Any sampling performed.
- Signatures of the persons performing and directly supervising or checking each critical step in the operation.
- In-process and laboratory test results.
- Actual yield at appropriate phases or times.
- Description of packaging and label for intermediate or API.
- Representative label of API or intermediate if made commercially available.
- Any deviation noted, its evaluation, investigation conducted (if appropriate) or reference to that investigation if stored separately.
- Results of release testing.

Written procedures should be established and followed for investigating critical deviations or the failure of a batch of intermediate or API to meet specifications. The investigation should extend to other batches that may have been associated with the specific failure or deviation.

F. Laboratory Control Records (6.6)

Laboratory control records should include complete data derived from all tests conducted to ensure compliance with established specifications and standards, including examinations and assays, as follows:

- A description of samples received for testing, including the material name or source, batch number or other distinctive code, date sample was taken, and, where appropriate, the quantity and date the sample was received for testing.
- A statement of or reference to each test method used.
- A statement of the weight or measure of sample used for each test as described by the method; data on or cross-reference to the preparation and testing of reference standards, reagents and standard solutions.
- A complete record of all raw data generated during each test, in addition to graphs, charts and spectra from laboratory instrumentation, properly identified to show the specific material and batch tested.

- A record of all calculations performed in connection with the test, including, for example, units of measure, conversion factors, and equivalency factors.
- A statement of the test results and how they compare with established acceptance criteria
- The signature of the person who performed each test and the date(s) the tests were performed
- The date and signature of a second person showing that the original records have been reviewed for accuracy, completeness, and compliance with established standards

Complete records should also be maintained for :

- Any modifications to an established analytical method
- Periodic calibration of laboratory instruments, apparatus, gauges, and recording devices
- All stability testing performed on APIs
- Out-of-specification (OOS) investigations

G. Batch Production Record Review (6.7)

Written procedures should be established and followed for the review and approval of batch production and laboratory control records, including packaging and labeling, to determine compliance of the intermediate or API with established specifications before a batch is released or distributed.

Batch production and laboratory control records of critical process steps should be reviewed and approved by the quality unit(s) before an API batch is released or distributed. Production and laboratory control records of noncritical process steps can be reviewed by qualified production personnel or other units following procedures approved by the quality unit(s).

All deviation, investigation, and OOS reports should be reviewed as part of the batch record review before the batch is released.

The quality unit(s) can delegate to the production unit the responsibility and authority for release of intermediates, except for those shipped outside the control of the manufacturing company.

VII. MATERIALS MANAGEMENT (7)

A. General Controls (7.1)

There should be written procedures describing the receipt, identification, quarantine, storage, handling, sampling, testing, and approval or rejection of materials.

Manufacturers of intermediates and/or APIs should have a system for evaluating the suppliers of critical materials.

Materials should be purchased against an agreed specification, from a supplier, or suppliers, approved by the quality unit(s).

If the supplier of a critical material is not the manufacturer of that material, the name and address of that manufacturer should be known by the intermediate and/or API manufacturer.

Changing the source of supply of critical raw materials should be treated according to Section 13, Change Control.

B. Receipt and Quarantine (7.2)

Upon receipt and before acceptance, each container or grouping of containers of materials should be examined visually for correct labeling (including correlation between the name used by the supplier and the in-house name, if these are different), container damage, broken seals and evidence of tampering or contamination. Materials should be held under quarantine until they have been sampled, examined, or tested, as appropriate, and released for use.

Before incoming materials are mixed with existing stocks (e.g., solvents or stocks in silos), they should be identified as correct, tested, if appropriate, and released. Procedures should be available to prevent discharging incoming materials wrongly into the existing stock.

If bulk deliveries are made in nondedicated tankers, there should be assurance of no cross-contamination from the tanker. Means of providing this assurance could include one or more of the following :

- certificate of cleaning
- testing for trace impurities
- audit of the supplier

Large storage containers and their attendant manifolds, filling, and discharge lines should be appropriately identified.

Each container or grouping of containers (batches) of materials should be assigned and identified with a distinctive code, batch, or receipt number. This number should be used in recording the disposition of each batch. A system should be in place to identify the status of each batch.

C. Sampling and Testing of Incoming Production Materials (7.3)

At least one test to verify the identity of each batch of material should be conducted, with the exception of the materials described below. A *supplier's certificate of analysis* can be used in place of performing other tests, provided that the manufacturer has a system in place to evaluate suppliers.

Supplier approval should include an evaluation that provides adequate evidence (e.g., past quality history) that the manufacturer can consistently provide material meeting specifications. Complete analyses should be conducted on at least three batches before reducing in-house testing. However, as a minimum, a complete analysis should be performed at appropriate intervals and compared with the certificates of analysis. Reliability of certificates of analysis should be checked at regular intervals.

Processing aids, hazardous or highly toxic raw materials, other special materials, or materials transferred to another unit within the company's control do not need to be tested if the manufacturer's certificate of analysis is obtained, showing that these raw materials conform to established specifications. Visual examination of containers, labels, and recording of batch numbers should help in establishing the identity of these materials. The lack of on-site testing for these materials should be justified and documented.

Samples should be representative of the batch of material from which they are taken. Sampling methods should specify the number of containers to be sampled, which part of the container to sample, and the amount of material to be taken from each container. The number of containers to sample and the sample size should be based on a sampling plan that takes into consideration the criticality of the material, material variability, past quality history of the supplier, and the quantity needed for analysis.

Sampling should be conducted at defined locations and by procedures designed to prevent contamination of the material sampled and contamination of other materials.

Containers from which samples are withdrawn should be opened carefully and subsequently reclosed. They should be marked to indicate that a sample has been taken.

D. Storage (7.4)

Materials should be handled and stored in a manner to prevent degradation, contamination, and cross-contamination.

Materials stored in fiber drums, bags, or boxes should be stored off the floor and, when appropriate, suitably spaced to permit cleaning and inspection.

Materials should be stored under conditions and for a period that have no adverse effect on their quality, and should normally be controlled so that the oldest stock is used first.

Certain materials in suitable containers can be stored outdoors, provided identifying labels remain legible and containers are appropriately cleaned before opening and use.

Rejected materials should be identified and controlled under a quarantine system designed to prevent their unauthorized use in manufacturing.

E. Re-evaluation (7.5)

Materials should be re-evaluated, as appropriate, to determine their suitability for use (e.g., after prolonged storage or exposure to heat or humidity).

VIII. PRODUCTION AND IN-PROCESS CONTROLS (8)

A. Production Operations (8.1)

Raw materials for intermediate and API manufacturing should be weighed or measured under appropriate conditions that do not affect their suitability for use. Weighing and measuring devices should be of suitable accuracy for the intended use.

If a material is subdivided for later use in production operations, the container receiving the material should be suitable and should be so identified that the following information is available:

- Material name and/or item code
- Receiving or control number
- Weight or measure of material in the new container
- Re-evaluation or retest date if appropriate

Critical weighing, measuring, or subdividing operations should be witnessed or subjected to an equivalent control. Prior to use, production personnel should verify that the materials are those specified in the batch record for the intended intermediate or API.

Other critical activities should be witnessed or subjected to an equivalent control.

Actual yields should be compared with expected yields at designated steps in the production process. Expected yields with appropriate ranges should be established based on previous laboratory, pilot scale, or manufacturing data. Deviations in yield associated with critical process steps should be investigated to determine their impact or potential impact on the resulting quality of affected batches.

Any deviation should be documented and explained. Any critical deviation should be investigated.

The processing status of major units of equipment should be indicated either on the individual units of equipment or by appropriate documentation, computer control systems, or alternative means.

Materials to be reprocessed or reworked should be appropriately controlled to prevent unauthorized use.

B. Time Limits (8.2)

If time limits are specified in the master production instruction (see 6.40), these time limits should be met to ensure the quality of intermediates and APIs. Deviations should be documented and evaluated. Time limits may be inappropriate when processing to a target value (e.g., pH adjustment, hydrogenation, drying to predetermined specification) because completion of reactions or processing steps are determined by in-process sampling and testing.

Intermediates held for further processing should be stored under appropriate conditions to ensure their suitability for use.

C. In-process Sampling and Controls (8.3)

Written procedures should be established to monitor the progress and control the performance of processing steps that cause variability in the quality characteristics of intermediates and APIs. In-process controls and their acceptance criteria should be defined based on the information gained during the developmental stage or from historical data.

The acceptance criteria and type and extent of testing can depend on the nature of the intermediate or API being manufactured, the reaction or process step being conducted, and the degree to which the process introduces variability in the product's quality. Less stringent in-process controls may be appropriate in early processing steps, whereas tighter controls may be appropriate for later processing steps (e.g., isolation and purification steps).

Critical in-process controls (and critical process monitoring), including control points and methods, should be stated in writing and approved by the quality unit(s).

In-process controls can be performed by qualified production department personnel and the process adjusted without prior quality unit(s) approval if the adjustments are made within pre-established limits approved by the quality unit(s). All tests and results should be fully documented as part of the batch record.

Written procedures should describe the sampling methods for in-process materials, intermediates, and APIs. Sampling plans and procedures should be based on scientifically sound sampling practices.

In-process sampling should be conducted using procedures designed to prevent contamination of the sampled material and other intermediates or APIs. Procedures should be established to ensure the integrity of samples after collection.

Out-of-specification (OOS) investigations are not normally needed for in-process tests that are performed for the purpose of monitoring and/or adjusting the process.

D. Blending Batches of Intermediates or APIs (8.4)

For the purpose of this document, blending is defined as the process of combining materials within the same specification to produce a homogeneous intermediate or API. In-process mixing of fractions from single batches (e.g., collecting several centrifuge loads from a single crystallization batch) or combining fractions from several batches for further processing is considered to be part of the production process and is not considered to be blending.

Out-of-specification batches should not be blended with other batches for the purpose of meeting specifications. Each batch incorporated into the blend should have been manufactured using an established process and should have been individually tested and found to meet appropriate specifications prior to blending.

Acceptable blending operations include, but are not limited to :

- Blending of small batches to increase batch size
- Blending of tailings (i.e., relatively small quantities of isolated material) from batches of the same intermediate or API to form a single batch

Blending processes should be adequately controlled and documented, and the blended batch should be tested for conformance to established specifications, where appropriate.

The batch record of the blending process should allow traceability back to the individual batches that make up the blend.

Where physical attributes of the API are critical (e.g., APIs intended for use in solid oral dosage forms or suspensions), blending operations should be validated to show homogeneity of the combined batch. Validation should include testing of critical attributes (e.g., particle size distribution, bulk density, and tap density) that may be affected by the blending process.

If the blending could adversely affect stability, stability testing of the final blended batches should be performed.

The expiry or retest date of the blended batch should be based on the manufacturing date of the oldest tailings or batch in the blend.

E. Contamination Control (8.5)

Residual materials can be carried over into successive batches of the same intermediate or API if there is adequate control. Examples include residue adhering to the wall of a micronizer, residual layer of damp crystals remaining in a centrifuge bowl after discharge, and incomplete discharge of fluids or crystals from a processing vessel upon transfer of the material to the next step in the process. Such carryover should not result in the carryover of degradants or microbial contamination that may adversely alter the established API impurity profile.

Production operations should be conducted in a manner that prevents contamination of intermediates or APIs by other materials.

Precautions to avoid contamination should be taken when APIs are handled after purification.

IX. PACKAGING AND IDENTIFICATION LABELING OF APIs AND INTERMEDIATES (9)

A. General (9.1)

There should be written procedures describing the receipt, identification, quarantine, sampling, examination, and/or testing, release, and handling of packaging and labeling materials.

Packaging and labeling materials should conform to established specifications. Those that do not comply with such specifications should be rejected to prevent their use in operations for which they are unsuitable.

Records should be maintained for each shipment of labels and packaging materials showing receipt, examination, or testing, and whether accepted or rejected.

B. Packaging Materials (9.2)

Containers should provide adequate protection against deterioration or contamination of the intermediate or API that may occur during transportation and recommended storage.

Containers should be clean and, where indicated by the nature of the intermediate or API, sanitized to ensure that they are suitable for their intended use. These containers should not be reactive, additive, or absorptive so as to alter the quality of the intermediate or API beyond the specified limits.

If containers are reused, they should be cleaned in accordance with documented procedures, and all previous labels should be removed or defaced.

C. Label Issuance and Control (9.3)

Access to the label storage areas should be limited to authorized personnel.

Procedures should be established to reconcile the quantities of labels issued, used, and returned and to evaluate discrepancies found between the number of containers labeled and the number of labels issued. Such discrepancies should be investigated, and the investigation should be approved by the quality unit(s).

All excess labels bearing batch numbers or other batch-related printing should be destroyed. Returned labels should be maintained and stored in a manner that prevents mix-ups and provides proper identification.

Obsolete and out-dated labels should be destroyed.

Printing devices used to print labels for packaging operations should be controlled to ensure that all imprinting conforms to the print specified in the batch production record.

Printed labels issued for a batch should be carefully examined for proper identity and conformity to specifications in the master production record. The results of this examination should be documented.

A printed label representative of those used should be included in the batch production record.

D. Packaging and Labeling Operations (9.4)

There should be documented procedures designed to ensure that correct packaging materials and labels are used.

Labeling operations should be designed to prevent mix-ups. There should be physical or spatial separation from operations involving other intermediates or APIs.

Labels used on containers of intermediates or APIs should indicate the name or identifying code, batch number, and storage conditions when such information is critical to ensure the quality of intermediate or API.

If the intermediate or API is intended to be transferred outside the control of the manufacturer's material management system, the name and address of the manufacturer, quantity of contents, special transport conditions, and any special legal requirements should also be included on the label. For intermediates or APIs with an expiry date, the expiry date should be indicated on the label and certificate of analysis. For intermediates or APIs with a retest date, the retest date should be indicated on the label and/or certificate of analysis.

Packaging and labeling facilities should be inspected immediately before use to ensure that all materials not needed for the next packaging operation have been removed. This examination should be documented in the batch production records, the facility log, or other documentation system.

Packaged and labeled intermediates or APIs should be examined to ensure that containers and packages in the batch have the correct label. This examination should be part of the packaging operation. Results of these examinations should be recorded in the batch production or control records.

Intermediate or API containers that are transported outside of the manufacturer's control should be sealed in a manner such that, if the seal is breached or missing, the recipient will be alerted to the possibility that the contents may have been altered.

X. STORAGE AND DISTRIBUTION (10)

A. Warehousing Procedures (10.1)

Facilities should be available for the storage of all materials under appropriate conditions (e.g., controlled temperature and humidity when necessary). Records should be maintained of these conditions if they are critical for the maintenance of material characteristics.

Unless there is an alternative system to prevent the unintentional or unauthorized use of quarantined, rejected, returned, or recalled materials, separate storage areas should be assigned for their temporary storage until the decision as to their future use has been made.

B. Distribution Procedures (10.2)

APIs and intermediates should only be released for distribution to third parties after they have been released by the quality unit(s). APIs and intermediates can be transferred under quarantine to another unit under the company's control when authorized by the quality unit(s) and if appropriate controls and documentation are in place.

APIs and intermediates should be transported in a manner that does not adversely affect their quality.

Special transport or storage conditions for an API or intermediate should be stated on the label.

The manufacturer should ensure that the contract acceptor (contractor) for transportation of the API or intermediate knows and follows the appropriate transport and storage conditions.

A system should be in place by which the distribution of each batch of intermediate and/or API can be readily determined to permit its recall.

XI. LABORATORY CONTROLS (11)

A. General Controls (11.1)

The independent quality unit(s) should have at its disposal adequate laboratory facilities.

There should be documented procedures describing sampling, testing, approval, or rejection of materials and recording and storage of laboratory data. Laboratory records should be maintained in accordance with Section 6.6.

All specifications, sampling plans, and test procedures should be scientifically sound and appropriate to ensure that raw materials, intermediates, APIs, and labels and packaging materials conform to established standards of quality and/or purity. Specifications and test procedures should be consistent with those included in the registration/filing. There can be specifications in addition to those in the registration/filing. Specifications, sampling plans, and test procedures, including changes to them, should be drafted by the appropriate organizational unit and reviewed and approved by the quality unit(s).

Appropriate specifications should be established for APIs in accordance with accepted standards and consistent with the manufacturing process. The specifications should include control of impurities (e.g., organic impurities, inorganic impurities, and residual solvents). If the API has a specification for microbiological purity, appropriate action limits for total microbial counts and objectionable organisms should be established and met. If the API has a specification for endotoxins, appropriate action limits should be established and met.

Laboratory controls should be followed and documented at the time of performance. Any departures from the above-described procedures should be documented and explained.

Any out-of-specification result obtained should be investigated and documented according to a procedure. This procedure should include analysis of the data, assessment of whether a significant problem exists, allocation of the tasks for corrective actions, and conclusions. Any resampling and/or retesting after OOS results should be performed according to a documented procedure.

Reagents and standard solutions should be prepared and labeled following written procedures. *Use by* dates should be applied, as appropriate, for analytical reagents or standard solutions.

Primary reference standards should be obtained, as appropriate, for the manufacture of APIs. The source of each primary reference standard should be documented. Records should be maintained of each primary reference standard's storage and use in accordance with the supplier's recommendations. Primary reference standards obtained from an officially recognized source are normally used without testing if stored under conditions consistent with the supplier's recommendations.

Where a primary reference standard is not available from an officially recognized source, an *in-house primary standard* should be established. Appropriate testing should be performed to establish fully the identity and purity of the primary reference standard. Appropriate documentation of this testing should be maintained.

Secondary reference standards should be appropriately prepared, identified, tested, approved, and stored. The suitability of each batch of secondary reference standard should be determined prior to first use by comparing against a primary reference standard. Each batch of secondary reference standard should be periodically requalified in accordance with a written protocol.

B. Testing of Intermediates and APIs (11.2)

For each batch of intermediate and API, appropriate laboratory tests should be conducted to determine conformance to specifications.

An impurity profile describing the identified and unidentified impurities present in a typical batch produced by a specific controlled production process should normally be established for each API. The impurity profile should include the identity or some qualitative analytical designation (e.g., retention time), the range of each impurity observed, and classification of each identified impurity (e.g., inorganic, organic, solvent). The impurity profile is normally dependent upon the production process and origin of the API. Impurity profiles are normally not necessary for APIs from herbal or animal tissue origin. Biotechnology considerations are covered in ICH guidance Q6B.

The impurity profile should be compared at appropriate intervals against the impurity profile in the regulatory submission or compared against historical data to detect changes to the API resulting from modifications in raw materials, equipment operating parameters, or the production process.

Appropriate microbiological tests should be conducted on each batch of intermediate and API where microbial quality is specified.

C. Validation of Analytical Procedures - See Section 12. (11.3)

D. Certificates of Analysis (11.4)

Authentic certificates of analysis should be issued for each batch of intermediate or API on request.

Information on the name of the intermediate or API including, where appropriate, its grade, the batch number, and the date of release should be provided on the certificate of analysis. For intermediates or APIs with an expiry date, the expiry date should be provided on the label and certificate of analysis. For intermediates or APIs with a retest date, the retest date should be indicated on the label and/or certificate of analysis.

The certificate should list each test performed in accordance with compendial or customer requirements, including the acceptance limits, and the numerical results obtained (if test results are numerical).

Certificates should be dated and signed by authorized personnel of the quality unit(s) and should show the name, address, and telephone number of the original manufacturer. Where the analysis has been carried out by a repacker or reprocessor, the certificate of analysis should show the name, address, and telephone number of the repacker/ reprocessor and reference the name of the original manufacturer.

If new certificates are issued by or on behalf of repackers/ reprocessors, agents or brokers, these certificates should show the name, address and telephone number of the laboratory that performed the analysis. They should also contain a reference to the name and address of the original manufacturer and to the original batch certificate, a copy of which should be attached.

E. Stability Monitoring of APIs (11.5)

A documented, on-going testing program should be established to monitor the stability characteristics of APIs, and the results should be used to confirm appropriate storage conditions and retest or expiry dates.

The test procedures used in stability testing should be validated and be stability indicating.

Stability samples should be stored in containers that simulate the market container. For example, if the API is marketed in bags within fiber drums, stability samples can be packaged in bags of the same material and in small-scale drums of similar or identical material composition to the market drums.

Normally, the first three commercial production batches should be placed on the stability monitoring program to confirm the retest or expiry date. However, where data from previous studies show that the API is expected to remain stable for at least 2 years, fewer than three batches can be used.

Thereafter, at least one batch per year of API manufactured (unless none is produced that year) should be added to the stability monitoring program and tested at least annually to confirm the stability.

For APIs with short shelf-lives, testing should be done more frequently. For example, for those biotechnological/biologic and other APIs with shelf-lives of one year or less, stability samples should be obtained and should be tested monthly for the first 3 months, and at 3-month intervals after that. When data exist that confirm that the stability of the API is not compromised, elimination of specific test intervals (e.g., 9-month testing) can be considered.

Where appropriate, the stability storage conditions should be consistent with the ICH guidances on stability.

F. Expiry and Retest Dating (11.6)

When an intermediate is intended to be transferred outside the control of the manufacturer's material management system and an expiry or retest date is assigned, supporting stability information should be available (e.g., published data, test results).

An API expiry or retest date should be based on an evaluation of data derived from stability studies. Common practice is to use a retest date, not an expiration date.

Preliminary API expiry or retest dates can be based on pilot scale batches if (1) the pilot batches employ a method of manufacture and procedure that simulates the final process to be used on a commercial manufacturing scale and (2) the quality of the API represents the material to be made on a commercial scale.

A representative sample should be taken for the purpose of performing a retest.

G. Reserve/Retention Samples (11.7)

The packaging and holding of reserve samples is for the purpose of potential future evaluation of the quality of batches of API and not for future stability testing purposes.

Appropriately identified reserve samples of each API batch should be retained for 1 year after the expiry date of the batch assigned by the manufacturer, or for 3 years after distribution of the batch, whichever is longer. For APIs with retest dates, similar reserve samples should be retained for 3 years after the batch is completely distributed by the manufacturer.

The reserve sample should be stored in the same packaging system in which the API is stored or in one that is equivalent to or more protective than the marketed packaging system. Sufficient quantities should be retained to conduct at least two full compendial analyses or, when there is no pharmacopoeial monograph, two full specification analyses.

XII. VALIDATION (12)

A. Validation Policy (12.1)

The company's overall policy, intentions, and approach to validation, including the validation of production processes, cleaning procedures, analytical methods, in-process control test procedures, computerized systems, and persons responsible for design, review, approval, and documentation of each validation phase, should be documented.

The critical parameters/attributes should normally be identified during the development stage or from historical data, and the necessary ranges for the reproducible operation should be defined. This should include :

- Defining the API in terms of its critical product attributes.
- Identifying process parameters that could affect the critical quality attributes of the API.
- Determining the range for each critical process parameter expected to be used during routine manufacturing and process control.

Validation should extend to those operations determined to be critical to the quality and purity of the API.

B. Validation Documentation (12.2)

A written validation protocol should be established that specifies how validation of a particular process will be conducted. The protocol should be reviewed and approved by the quality unit(s) and other designated units.

The validation protocol should specify critical process steps and acceptance criteria as well as the type of validation to be conducted (e.g., retrospective, prospective, concurrent) and the number of process runs.

A validation report that cross-references the validation protocol should be prepared, summarizing the results obtained, commenting on any deviations observed, and drawing the appropriate conclusions, including recommending changes to correct deficiencies.

Any variations from the validation protocol should be documented with appropriate justification.

C. Qualification (12.3)

Before initiating process validation activities, appropriate qualification of critical equipment and ancillary systems should be completed. Qualification is usually carried out by conducting the following activities, individually or combined :

- *Design Qualification (DQ):* documented verification that the proposed design of the facilities, equipment, or systems is suitable for the intended purpose.
- *Installation Qualification (IQ) :* documented verification that the equipment or systems, as installed or modified, comply with the approved design, the manufacturer's recommendations and/or user requirements.

- *Operational Qualification (OQ) :* documented verification that the equipment or systems, as installed or modified, perform as intended throughout the anticipated operating ranges
- *Performance Qualification (PQ) :* documented verification that the equipment and ancillary systems, as connected together, can perform effectively and reproducibly based on the approved process method and specifications

D. Approaches to Process Validation (12.4)

Process Validation (PV) is the documented evidence that the process, operated within established parameters, can perform effectively and reproducibly to produce an intermediate or API meeting its predetermined specifications and quality attributes.

There are three approaches to validation. Prospective validation is the preferred approach, but there are situations where the other approaches can be used. These approaches and their applicability are discussed here.

Prospective validation should normally be performed for all API processes as defined in 12.1. Prospective validation of an API process should be completed before the commercial distribution of the final drug product manufactured from that API.

Concurrent validation can be conducted when data from replicate production runs are unavailable because only a limited number of API batches have been produced, API batches are produced infrequently, or API batches are produced by a validated process that has been modified. Prior to the completion of concurrent validation, batches can be released and used in final drug product for commercial distribution based on thorough monitoring and testing of the API batches.

An exception can be made for retrospective validation of well-established processes that have been used without significant changes to API quality due to changes in raw materials, equipment, systems, facilities, or the production process. This validation approach may be used where:

1. Critical quality attributes and critical process parameters have been identified.
2. Appropriate in-process acceptance criteria and controls have been established.

3. There have not been significant process/product failures attributable to causes other than operator error or equipment failures unrelated to equipment suitability.
4. Impurity profiles have been established for the existing API

Batches selected for retrospective validation should be representative of all batches produced during the review period, including any batches that failed to meet specifications, and should be sufficient in number to demonstrate process consistency. Retained samples can be tested to obtain data to retrospectively validate the process.

E. Process Validation Program (12.5)

The number of process runs for validation should depend on the complexity of the process or the magnitude of the process change being considered. For prospective and concurrent validation, three consecutive successful production batches should be used as a guide, but there may be situations where additional process runs are warranted to prove consistency of the process (e.g., complex API processes or API processes with prolonged completion times). For retrospective validation, generally data from 10 to 30 consecutive batches should be examined to assess process consistency, but fewer batches can be examined if justified.

Critical process parameters should be controlled and monitored during process validation studies. Process parameters unrelated to quality, such as variables controlled to minimize energy consumption or equipment use, need not be included in the process validation.

Process validation should confirm that the impurity profile for each API is within the limits specified. The impurity profile should be comparable to, or better than, historical data and, where applicable, the profile determined during process development or for batches used for pivotal clinical and toxicological studies.

F. Periodic Review of Validated Systems (12.6)

Systems and processes should be periodically evaluated to verify that they are still operating in a valid manner. Where no significant changes have been made to the system or process, and a quality review confirms that the system or process is consistently producing material meeting its specifications, there is normally no need for revalidation.

G. Cleaning Validation (12.7)

Cleaning procedures should normally be validated. In general, cleaning validation should be directed to situations or process steps where contamination or carryover of materials poses the greatest risk to API quality. For example, in early production it may be unnecessary to validate equipment cleaning procedures where residues are removed by subsequent purification steps.

Validation of cleaning procedures should reflect actual equipment usage patterns. If various APIs or intermediates are manufactured in the same equipment and the equipment is cleaned by the same process, a representative intermediate or API can be selected for cleaning validation. This selection should be based on the solubility and difficulty of cleaning and the calculation of residue limits based on potency, toxicity, and stability.

The cleaning validation protocol should describe the equipment to be cleaned, procedures, materials, acceptable cleaning levels, parameters to be monitored and controlled, and analytical methods. The protocol should also indicate the type of samples to be obtained and how they are collected and labeled.

Sampling should include swabbing, rinsing, or alternative methods (e.g., direct extraction), as appropriate, to detect both insoluble and soluble residues. The sampling methods used should be capable of quantitatively measuring levels of residues remaining on the equipment surfaces after cleaning. Swab sampling may be impractical when product contact surfaces are not easily accessible due to equipment design and/or process limitations (e.g., inner surfaces of hoses, transfer pipes, reactor tanks with small ports or handling toxic materials, and small intricate equipment such as micronizers and microfluidizers).

Validated analytical methods having sensitivity to detect residues or contaminants should be used. The detection limit for each analytical method should be sufficiently sensitive to detect the established acceptable level of the residue or contaminant. The method's attainable recovery level should be established. Residue limits should be practical, achievable, verifiable, and based on the most deleterious residue. Limits can be established based on the minimum known pharmacological, toxicological, or physiological activity of the API or its most deleterious component.

Equipment cleaning/sanitation studies should address microbiological and endotoxin contamination for those processes where there is a need to reduce total microbiological count or endotoxins in the API, or other processes where such contamination could be of concern (e.g., non-sterile APIs used to manufacture sterile products).

Cleaning procedures should be monitored at appropriate intervals after validation to ensure that these procedures are effective when used during routine production. Equipment cleanliness can be monitored by analytical testing and visual examination, where feasible. Visual inspection can allow detection of gross contamination concentrated in small areas that could otherwise go undetected by sampling and/or analysis.

H. Validation of Analytical Methods (12.8)

Analytical methods should be validated unless the method employed is included in the relevant pharmacopoeia or other recognized standard reference. The suitability of all testing methods used should nonetheless be verified under actual conditions of use and documented.

Methods should be validated to include consideration of characteristics included within the ICH guidances on validation of analytical methods. The degree of analytical validation performed should reflect the purpose of the analysis and the stage of the API production process.

Appropriate qualification of analytical equipment should be considered before initiating validation of analytical methods.

Complete records should be maintained of any modification of a validated analytical method. Such records should include the reason for the modification and appropriate data to verify that the modification produces results that are as accurate and reliable as the established method.

XIII. CHANGE CONTROL (13)

A formal change control system should be established to evaluate all changes that could affect the production and control of the intermediate or API.

Written procedures should provide for the identification, documentation, appropriate review, and approval of changes in raw materials, specifications, analytical methods, facilities, support systems, equipment (including computer hardware), processing steps, labeling and packaging materials, and computer software.

Any proposals for GMP relevant changes should be drafted, reviewed, and approved by the appropriate organizational units and reviewed and approved by the quality unit(s).

The potential impact of the proposed change on the quality of the intermediate or API should be evaluated. A classification procedure may help in determining the level of testing, validation, and documentation needed to justify changes to a validated process. Changes can be classified (e.g., as minor or major) depending on the nature and extent of the changes, and the effects these changes may impart on the process. Scientific judgment should determine what additional testing and validation studies are appropriate to justify a change in a validated process.

When implementing approved changes, measures should be taken to ensure that all documents affected by the changes are revised.

After the change has been implemented, there should be an evaluation of the first batches produced or tested under the change.

The potential for critical changes to affect established retest or expiry dates should be evaluated. If necessary, samples of the intermediate or API produced by the modified process can be placed on an accelerated stability program and/or can be added to the stability monitoring program.

Current dosage form manufacturers should be notified of changes from established production and process control procedures that can affect the quality of the API.

XIV. REJECTION AND RE-USE OF MATERIALS (14)

A. Rejection (14.1)

Intermediates and APIs failing to meet established specifications should be identified as such and quarantined. These intermediates or APIs can be reprocessed or reworked as described below. The final disposition of rejected materials should be recorded.

B. Reprocessing (14.2)

Introducing an intermediate or API, including one that does not conform to standards or specifications, back into the process and reprocessing by repeating a crystallization step or other appropriate chemical or physical manipulation steps (e.g., distillation, filtration, chromatography, milling) that are part of the established manufacturing process is generally considered acceptable. However, if such reprocessing is used for a majority of batches, such reprocessing should be included as part of the standard manufacturing process.

Continuation of a process step after an in-process control test has shown that the step is incomplete is considered to be part of the normal process. This is not considered to be reprocessing.

Introducing unreacted material back into a process and repeating a chemical reaction is considered to be reprocessing unless it is part of the established process. Such reprocessing should be preceded by careful evaluation to ensure that the quality of the intermediate or API is not adversely affected due to the potential formation of by-products and over-reacted materials.

C. Reworking (14.3)

Before a decision is taken to rework batches that do not conform to established standards or specifications, an investigation into the reason for nonconformance should be performed.

Batches that have been reworked should be subjected to appropriate evaluation, testing, stability testing if warranted, and documentation to show that the reworked product is of equivalent quality to that produced by the original process. Concurrent validation is often the appropriate validation approach for rework procedures. This allows a protocol to define the rework procedure, how it will be carried out, and the expected results. If there is only one batch to be reworked, a report can be written and the batch released once it is found to be acceptable.

Procedures should provide for comparing the impurity profile of each reworked batch against batches manufactured by the established process. Where routine analytical methods are inadequate to characterize the reworked batch, additional methods should be used.

D. Recovery of Materials and Solvents (14.4)

Recovery (e.g., from mother liquor or filtrates) of reactants, intermediates, or the API is considered acceptable, provided that approved procedures exist for the recovery and the recovered materials meet specifications suitable for their intended use.

Solvents can be recovered and reused in the same processes or in different processes, provided that the recovery procedures are controlled and monitored to ensure that solvents meet appropriate standards before reuse or commingling with other approved materials.

Fresh and recovered solvents and reagents can be combined if adequate testing has shown their suitability for all manufacturing processes in which they may be used.

The use of recovered solvents, mother liquors, and other recovered materials should be adequately documented.

E. Returns (14.5)

Returned intermediates or APIs should be identified as such and quarantined.

If the conditions under which returned intermediates or APIs have been stored or shipped before or during their return or the condition of their containers casts doubt on their quality, the returned intermediates or APIs should be reprocessed, reworked, or destroyed, as appropriate.

Records of returned intermediates or APIs should be maintained. For each return, documentation should include:

- Name and address of the consignee
- Intermediate or API, batch number, and quantity returned
- Reason for return
- Use or disposal of the returned intermediate or API

XV. COMPLAINTS AND RECALLS (15)

All quality-related complaints, whether received orally or in writing, should be recorded and investigated according to a written procedure.

Complaint records should include :

- Name and address of complainant
- Name (and, where appropriate, title) and phone number of person submitting the complaint
- Complaint nature (including name and batch number of the API)
- Date complaint is received
- Action initially taken (including dates and identity of person taking the action);
- Any follow-up action taken
- Response provided to the originator of complaint (including date response sent)
- Final decision on intermediate or API batch or lot

Records of complaints should be retained to evaluate trends, product-related frequencies, and severity with a view to taking additional, and if appropriate, immediate corrective action.

There should be a written procedure that defines the circumstances under which a recall of an intermediate or API should be considered.

The recall procedure should designate who should be involved in evaluating the information, how a recall should be initiated, who should be informed about the recall, and how the recalled material should be treated.

In the event of a serious or potentially life-threatening situation, local, national, and/or international authorities should be informed and their advice sought.

XVI. CONTRACT MANUFACTURERS (INCLUDING LABORATORIES) (16)

All contract manufacturers (including laboratories) should comply with the GMP defined in this guidance. Special consideration should be given to the prevention of cross-contamination and to maintaining traceability.

Companies should evaluate any contractors (including laboratories) to ensure GMP compliance of the specific operations occurring at the contractor sites.

There should be a written and approved contract or formal agreement between a company and its contractors that defines in detail the GMP responsibilities, including the quality measures, of each party.

A contract should permit a company to audit its contractor's facilities for compliance with GMP.

Where subcontracting is allowed, a contractor should not pass to a third party any of the work entrusted to it under the contract without the company's prior evaluation and approval of the arrangements.

Manufacturing and laboratory records should be kept at the site where the activity occurs and be readily available.

Changes in the process, equipment, test methods, specifications, or other contractual requirements should not be made unless the contract giver is informed and approves the changes.

XVII. AGENTS, BROKERS, TRADERS, DISTRIBUTORS, REPACKERS, AND RELABELLERS (17)

A. Applicability (17.1)

This section applies to any party other than the original manufacturer who may trade and/or take possession, repack, relabel, manipulate, distribute, or store an API or intermediate.

All agents, brokers, traders, distributors, repackers, and relabelers should comply with GMP as defined in this guidance.

B. Traceability of Distributed APIs and Intermediates (17.2)

Agents, brokers, traders, distributors, repackers, or relabelers should maintain complete traceability of APIs and intermediates that they distribute. Documents that should be retained and available include :

- Identity of original manufacturer
- Address of original manufacturer
- Purchase orders
- Bills of lading (transportation documentation)
- Receipt documents
- Name or designation of API or intermediate
- Manufacturer's batch number
- Transportation and distribution records
- All authentic Certificates of Analysis, including those of the original manufacturer
- Retest or expiry date

C. Quality Management (17.3)

Agents, brokers, traders, distributors, repackers, or relabelers should establish, document and implement an effective system of managing quality, as specified in Section 2.

D. Repackaging, Relabeling, and Holding of APIs and Intermediates (17.4)

Repackaging, relabeling, and holding APIs and intermediates should be performed under appropriate GMP controls, as stipulated in this guidance, to avoid mix-ups and loss of API or intermediate identity or purity.

Repackaging should be conducted under appropriate environmental conditions to avoid contamination and cross-contamination.

E. Stability (17.5)

Stability studies to justify assigned expiration or retest dates should be conducted if the API or intermediate is repackaged in a different type of container than that used by the API or intermediate manufacturer.

F. Transfer of Information (17.6)

Agents, brokers, distributors, repackers, or relabelers should transfer all quality or regulatory information received from an API or intermediate manufacturer to the customer, and from the customer to the API or intermediate manufacturer.

The agent, broker, trader, distributor, repacker, or relabeler who supplies the API or intermediate to the customer should provide the name of the original API or intermediate manufacturer and the batch number(s) supplied.

The agent should also provide the identity of the original API or intermediate manufacturer to regulatory authorities upon request. The original manufacturer can respond to the regulatory authority directly or through its authorized agents, depending on the legal relationship between the authorized agents and the original API or intermediate manufacturer. (In this context authorized refers to *authorized* by the manufacturer.)

The specific guidance for certificate of analysis included in Section 11.4 should be met.

G. Handling of Complaints and Recalls (17.7)

Agents, brokers, traders, distributors, repackers, or relabelers should maintain records of complaints and recalls, as specified in Section 15, for all complaints and recalls that come to their attention.

If the situation warrants, the agents, brokers, traders, distributors, repackers, or relabelers should review the complaint with the original API or intermediate manufacturer to determine whether any further action, either with other customers who may have received this API or intermediate or with the regulatory authority, or both, should be initiated. The investigation into the cause for the complaint or recall should be conducted and documented by the appropriate party.

Where a complaint is referred to the original API or intermediate manufacturer, the record maintained by the agents, brokers, traders, distributors, repackers, or relabelers should include any response received from the original API or intermediate manufacturer (including date and information provided).

H. Handling of Returns (17.8)

Returns should be handled as specified in Section 14.5. The agents, brokers, traders, distributors, repackers, or relabelers should maintain documentation of returned APIs and intermediates.

XVIII. SPECIFIC GUIDANCE FOR APIs MANUFACTURED BY CELL CULTURE/FERMENTATION (18)

A. General (18.1)

Section 18 is intended to address specific controls for APIs or intermediates manufactured by cell culture or fermentation using natural or recombinant organisms and that have not been covered adequately in the previous sections. It is not intended to be a stand-alone section.

In general, the GMP principles in the other sections of this document apply. Note that the principles of fermentation for *classical* processes for production of small molecules and for processes using recombinant and nonrecombinant organisms for production of proteins and/or polypeptides are the same, although the degree of control will differ. Where practical, this section will address these differences. In general, the degree of control for biotechnological processes used to produce proteins and polypeptides is greater than that for classical fermentation processes.

The term biotechnological process (biotech) refers to the use of cells or organisms that have been generated or modified by recombinant DNA, hybridoma, or other technology to produce APIs. The APIs produced by biotechnological processes normally consist of high molecular weight substances, such as proteins and polypeptides, for which specific guidance is given in this Section. Certain APIs of low molecular weight, such as antibiotics, amino acids, vitamins, and carbohydrates, can also be produced by recombinant DNA technology. The level of control for these types of APIs is similar to that employed for classical fermentation.

The term classical fermentation refers to processes that use microorganisms existing in nature and/or modified by conventional methods (e.g., irradiation or chemical mutagenesis) to produce APIs. APIs produced by classical fermentation are normally low molecular weight products such as antibiotics, amino acids, vitamins, and carbohydrates.

Production of APIs or intermediates from cell culture or fermentation involves biological processes such as cultivation of cells or extraction and purification of material from living organisms. Note that there may be additional process steps, such as physicochemical modification, that are part of the manufacturing process. The raw materials used (media, buffer components) may provide the potential for growth of microbiological contaminants. Depending on the source, method of preparation, and the intended use of the API or intermediate, control of bioburden, viral contamination, and/or endotoxins during manufacturing and monitoring of the process at appropriate stages may be necessary.

Appropriate controls should be established at all stages of manufacturing to ensure intermediate and/or API quality. While this guidance starts at the cell culture/fermentation step, prior steps (e.g., cell banking) should be performed under appropriate process controls. This guidance covers cell culture/fermentation from the point at which a vial of the cell bank is retrieved for use in manufacturing.

Appropriate equipment and environmental controls should be used to minimize the risk of contamination. The acceptance criteria for determining environmental quality and the frequency of monitoring should depend on the step in production and the production conditions (open, closed, or contained systems).

In general, process controls should take into account :

- Maintenance of the working cell bank (where appropriate).
- Proper inoculation and expansion of the culture.
- Control of the critical operating parameters during fermentation/ cell culture.
- Monitoring of the process for cell growth, viability (for most cell culture processes) and productivity, where appropriate.
- Harvest and purification procedures that remove cells, cellular debris and media components while protecting the intermediate or API from contamination (particularly of a microbiological nature) and from loss of quality
- Monitoring of bioburden and, where needed, endotoxin levels at appropriate stages of production.
- *Viral safety concerns as described in ICH guidance Q5A* Quality of Biotechnological Products: Viral Safety Evaluation of Biotechnology Products Derived from Cell Lines of Human or Animal Origin.

Where appropriate, the removal of media components, host cell proteins, other process-related impurities, product-related impurities and contaminants should be demonstrated.

B. Cell Bank Maintenance and Record Keeping (18.2)

Access to cell banks should be limited to authorized personnel.

Cell banks should be maintained under storage conditions designed to maintain viability and prevent contamination.

Records of the use of the vials from the cell banks and storage conditions should be maintained.

Where appropriate, cell banks should be periodically monitored to determine suitability for use.

See ICH guidance Q5D *Quality of Biotechnological Products : Derivation and Characterization of Cell Substrates Used for Production of Biotechnological/Biological Products* for a more complete discussion of cell banking.

C. Cell Culture/Fermentation (18.3)

Where cell substrates, media, buffers, and gases are to be added under aseptic conditions, closed or contained systems should be used where possible. If the inoculation of the initial vessel or subsequent transfers or additions (media, buffers) are performed in open vessels, there should be controls and procedures in place to minimize the risk of contamination.

Where the quality of the API can be affected by microbial contamination, manipulations using open vessels should be performed in a biosafety cabinet or similarly controlled environment.

Personnel should be appropriately gowned and take special precautions handling the cultures.

Critical operating parameters (for example temperature, pH, agitation rates, addition of gases, pressure) should be monitored to ensure consistency with the established process. Cell growth, viability (for most cell culture processes), and, where appropriate, productivity should also be monitored. Critical parameters will vary from one process to another, and for classical fermentation, certain parameters (cell viability, for example) may not need to be monitored.

Cell culture equipment should be cleaned and sterilized after use. As appropriate, fermentation equipment should be cleaned, sanitized, or sterilized.

Culture media should be sterilized before use, when necessary, to protect the quality of the API.

Appropriate procedures should be in place to detect contamination and determine the course of action to be taken. Procedures should be available to determine the impact of the contamination on the product and to decontaminate the equipment and return it to a condition to be used in subsequent batches. Foreign organisms observed during fermentation processes should be identified, as appropriate, and the effect of their presence on product quality should be assessed, if necessary. The results of such assessments should be taken into consideration in the disposition of the material produced.

Records of contamination events should be maintained.

Shared (multi-product) equipment may warrant additional testing after cleaning between product campaigns, as appropriate, to minimize the risk of cross-contamination.

D. Harvesting, Isolation and Purification (18.4)

Harvesting steps, either to remove cells or cellular components or to collect cellular components after disruption should be performed in equipment and areas designed to minimize the risk of contamination.

Harvest and purification procedures that remove or inactivate the producing organism, cellular debris and media components (while minimizing degradation, contamination, and loss of quality) should be adequate to ensure that the intermediate or API is recovered with consistent quality.

All equipment should be properly cleaned and, as appropriate, sanitized after use. Multiple successive batching without cleaning can be used if intermediate or API quality is not compromised.

If open systems are used, purification should be performed under environmental conditions appropriate for the preservation of product quality.

Additional controls, such as the use of dedicated chromatography resins or additional testing, may be appropriate if equipment is to be used for multiple products.

E. Viral Removal/Inactivation steps (18.5)

See ICH guidance Q5A *Quality of Biotechnological Products: Viral Safety Evaluation of Biotechnology Products Derived from Cell Lines of Human or Animal Origin* for more specific information.

Viral removal and viral inactivation steps are critical processing steps for some processes and should be performed within their validated parameters.

Appropriate precautions should be taken to prevent potential viral contamination from previral to postviral removal/inactivation steps. Therefore, open processing should be performed in areas that are separate from other processing activities and have separate air handling units.

The same equipment is not normally used for different purification steps. However, if the same equipment is to be used, the equipment should be appropriately cleaned and sanitized before reuse. Appropriate precautions should be taken to prevent potential virus carry-over (e.g., through equipment or environment) from previous steps.

XIX. APIs FOR USE IN CLINICAL TRIALS (19)

A. General (19.1)

Not all the controls in the previous sections of this guidance are appropriate for the manufacture of a new API for investigational use during its development. Section XIX (19) provides specific guidance unique to these circumstances.

The controls used in the manufacture of APIs for use in clinical trials should be consistent with the stage of development of the drug product incorporating the API. Process and test procedures should be flexible to provide for changes as knowledge of the process increases and clinical testing of a drug product progresses from pre-clinical stages through clinical stages. Once drug development reaches the stage where the API is produced for use in drug products intended for clinical trials, manufacturers should ensure that APIs are manufactured in suitable facilities using appropriate production and control procedures to ensure the quality of the API.

B. Quality (19.2)

Appropriate GMP concepts should be applied in the production of APIs for use in clinical trials with a suitable mechanism for approval of each batch.

A quality unit(s) independent from production should be established for the approval or rejection of each batch of API for use in clinical trials.

Some of the testing functions commonly performed by the quality unit(s) can be performed within other organizational units.

Quality measures should include a system for testing of raw materials, packaging materials, intermediates, and APIs.

Process and quality problems should be evaluated.

Labeling for APIs intended for use in clinical trials should be appropriately controlled and should identify the material as being for investigational use.

C. Equipment and Facilities (19.3)

During all phases of clinical development, including the use of small-scale facilities or laboratories to manufacture batches of APIs for use in clinical trials, procedures should be in place to ensure that equipment is calibrated, clean, and suitable for its intended use.

Procedures for the use of facilities should ensure that materials are handled in a manner that minimizes the risk of contamination and cross-contamination.

D. Control of Raw Materials (19.4)

Raw materials used in production of APIs for use in clinical trials should be evaluated by testing, or received with a supplier's analysis and subjected to identity testing. When a material is considered hazardous, a supplier's analysis should suffice.

In some instances, the suitability of a raw material can be determined before use based on acceptability in small-scale reactions (i.e., use testing) rather than on analytical testing alone.

E. Production (19.5)

The production of APIs for use in clinical trials should be documented in laboratory notebooks, batch records, or by other appropriate means. These documents should include information on the use of production materials, equipment, processing, and scientific observations.

Expected yields can be more variable and less defined than the expected yields used in commercial processes. Investigations into yield variations are not expected.

F. Validation (19.6)

Process validation for the production of APIs for use in clinical trials is normally inappropriate, where a single API batch is produced or where process changes during API development make batch replication difficult or inexact. The combination of controls, calibration, and, where appropriate, equipment qualification ensures API quality during this development phase.

Process validation should be conducted in accordance with Section 12 when batches are produced for commercial use, even when such batches are produced on a pilot or small scale.

G. Changes (19.7)

Changes are expected during development, as knowledge is gained and the production is scaled up. Every change in the production, specifications, or test procedures should be adequately recorded.

H. Laboratory Controls (19.8)

While analytical methods performed to evaluate a batch of API for clinical trials may not yet be validated, they should be scientifically sound.

A system for retaining reserve samples of all batches should be in place. This system should ensure that a sufficient quantity of each reserve sample is retained for an appropriate length of time after approval, termination, or discontinuation of an application.

Expiry and retest dating as defined in Section 11.6 applies to existing APIs used in clinical trials. For new APIs, Section 11.6 does not normally apply in early stages of clinical trials.

I. Documentation (19.9)

A system should be in place to ensure that information gained during the development and the manufacture of APIs for use in clinical trials is documented and available.

The development and implementation of the analytical methods used to support the release of a batch of API for use in clinical trials should be appropriately documented.

A system for retaining production and control records and documents should be used. This system should ensure that records and documents are retained for an appropriate length of time after the approval, termination, or discontinuation of an application.

XX GLOSSARY (20)

Acceptance Criteria : Numerical limits, ranges, or other suitable measures for acceptance of test results.

Active Pharmaceutical Ingredient (API) (or Drug Substance) : Any substance or mixture of substances intended to be used in the manufacture of a drug (medicinal) product and that, when used in the production of a drug, becomes an active ingredient of the drug product. Such substances are intended to furnish pharmacological activity or other direct effect in the diagnosis, cure, mitigation, treatment, or prevention of disease or to affect the structure and function of the body.

API Starting Material : A raw material, intermediate, or an API that is used in the production of an API and that is incorporated as a significant structural fragment into the structure of the API. An API starting material can be an article of commerce, a material purchased from one or more suppliers under contract or commercial agreement, or produced in-house. API starting materials are normally of defined chemical properties and structure.

Batch (or Lot) : A specific quantity of material produced in a process or series of processes so that it is expected to be homogeneous within specified limits. In the case of continuous production, a batch may correspond to a defined fraction of the production. The batch size can be defined either by a fixed quantity or by the amount produced in a fixed time interval.

Batch Number (or Lot Number) : A unique combination of numbers, letters, and/or symbols that identifies a batch (or lot) and from which the production and distribution history can be determined.

Bioburden : The level and type (e.g., objectionable or not) of microorganisms that can be present in raw materials, API starting materials, intermediates or APIs. Bioburden should not be considered contamination unless the levels have been exceeded or defined objectionable organisms have been detected.

Calibration : The demonstration that a particular instrument or device produces results within specified limits by comparison with results produced by a reference or traceable standard over an appropriate range of measurements.

Computer System : A group of hardware components and associated software designed and assembled to perform a specific function or group of functions.

Computerized System : A process or operation integrated with a computer system.

Contamination : The undesired introduction of impurities of a chemical or microbiological nature, or of foreign matter, into or onto a raw material, intermediate, or API during production, sampling, packaging, or repackaging, storage or transport.

Contract Manufacturer : A manufacturer who performs some aspect of manufacturing on behalf of the original manufacturer.

Critical : Describes a process step, process condition, test requirement, or other relevant parameter or item that must be controlled within predetermined criteria to ensure that the API meets its specification.

Cross-Contamination : Contamination of a material or product with another material or product.

Deviation : Departure from an approved instruction or established standard.

Drug (Medicinal) Product : The dosage form in the final immediate packaging intended for marketing. (Reference Q1A)

Drug Substance : See Active Pharmaceutical Ingredient.

Expiry Date (or Expiration Date) : The date placed on the container/ labels of an API designating the time during which the API is expected to remain within established shelf life specifications if stored under defined conditions and after which it should not be used.

Impurity : Any component present in the intermediate or API that is not the desired entity.

Impurity Profile : A description of the identified and unidentified impurities present in an API.

In-Process Control (or Process Control) : Checks performed during production to monitor and, if appropriate, to adjust the process and/or to ensure that the intermediate or API conforms to its specifications.

Intermediate : A material produced during steps of the processing of an API that undergoes further molecular change or purification before it becomes an API. Intermediates may or may not be isolated. (Note: this guidance only addresses those intermediates produced after the point that a company has defined as the point at which the production of the API begins.)

Lot : See Batch

Lot Number : *See* Batch Number

Manufacture : All operations of receipt of materials, production, packaging, repackaging, labeling, relabeling, quality control, release, storage, and distribution of APIs and related controls.

Material : A general term used to denote raw materials (starting materials, reagents, solvents), process aids, intermediates, APIs, and packaging and labeling materials.

Mother Liquor : The residual liquid that remains after the crystallization or isolation processes. A mother liquor may contain unreacted materials, intermediates, levels of the API, and/or impurities. It can be used for further processing.

Packaging Material : Any material intended to protect an intermediate or API during storage and transport.

Procedure : A documented description of the operations to be performed, the precautions to be taken, and measures to be applied directly or indirectly related to the manufacture of an intermediate or API.

Process Aids : Materials, excluding solvents, used as an aid in the manufacture of an intermediate or API that do not themselves participate in a chemical or biological reaction (e.g., filter aid, activated carbon).

Process Control : See ***In-Process Control.***

Production : All operations involved in the preparation of an API from receipt of materials through processing and packaging of the API.

Qualification : Action of proving and documenting that equipment or ancillary systems are properly installed, work correctly, and actually lead to the expected results. Qualification is part of validation, but the individual qualification steps alone do not constitute process validation.

Quality Assurance (QA) : The sum total of the organized arrangements made with the object of ensuring that all APIs are of the quality required for their intended use and that quality systems are maintained.

Quality Control (QC) : Checking or testing that specifications are met.

Quality Unit(s) : An organizational unit independent of production that fulfills both quality assurance and quality control responsibilities. This can be in the form of separate QA and QC units or a single individual or group, depending upon the size and structure of the organization.

Quarantine : The status of materials isolated physically or by other effective means pending a decision on their subsequent approval or rejection.

Raw Material : A general term used to denote starting materials, reagents, and solvents intended for use in the production of intermediates or APIs.

Reference Standard, Primary : A substance that has been shown by an extensive set of analytical tests to be authentic material that should be of high purity. This standard can be: (1) obtained from an officially recognized source, (2) prepared by independent synthesis, (3) obtained from existing production material of high purity, or (4) prepared by further purification of existing production material.

Reference Standard, Secondary : A substance of established quality and purity, as shown by comparison to a primary reference standard, used as a reference standard for routine laboratory analysis.

Reprocessing : Introducing an intermediate or API, including one that does not conform to standards or specifications, back into the process and repeating a crystallization step or other appropriate chemical or physical manipulation steps (e.g., distillation, filtration, chromatography, milling) that are part of the established manufacturing process. Continuation of a process step after an in-process control test has shown that the step is incomplete, is considered to be part of the normal process, and is not reprocessing.

Retest Date : The date when a material should be re-examined to ensure that it is still suitable for use.

Reworking : Subjecting an intermediate or API that does not conform to standards or specifications to one or more processing steps that are different from the established manufacturing process to obtain acceptable quality intermediate or API (e.g., recrystallizing with a different solvent).

Signature (signed) : See definition for signed.

Signed (signature) : The record of the individual who performed a particular action or review. This record can be initials, full handwritten signature, personal seal, or authenticated and secure electronic signature.

Solvent : An inorganic or organic liquid used as a vehicle for the preparation of solutions or suspensions in the manufacture of an intermediate or API.

Specification : A list of tests, references to analytical procedures, and appropriate acceptance criteria that are numerical limits, ranges, or other criteria for the test described. It establishes the set of criteria to which a material should conform to be considered acceptable for its intended use. *Conformance to specification* means that the material, when tested according to the listed analytical procedures, will meet the listed acceptance criteria.

Validation : A documented program that provides a high degree of assurance that a specific process, method, or system will consistently produce a result meeting predetermined acceptance criteria.

Validation Protocol : A written plan stating how validation will be conducted and defining acceptance criteria. For example, the protocol for a manufacturing process identifies processing equipment, critical process parameters and/or operating ranges, product characteristics, sampling, test data to be collected, number of validation runs, and acceptable test results.

Yield, Expected : The quantity of material or the percentage of theoretical yield anticipated at any appropriate phase of production based on previous laboratory, pilot scale, or manufacturing data.

Yield, Theoretical : The quantity that would be produced at any appropriate phase of production based upon the quantity of material to be used, in the absence of any loss or error in actual production.

Bibliography

1. *ISO 9000-3:1997,* Quality management and quality assurance standards— Part 3: Guidelines for the application of ISO 9001:1994 to the development, supply, installation and maintenance of computer software.
2. *1309004:2000,* Quality management systems —Guidelines for performance improvements.
3. *ISO 10005:1995,* Quality management — Guidelines for quality plans.
4. *ISO 10006:1997,* Quality management — Guidelines to quality In project management.
5. *ISO 10007:1995.* duality management—Guidelines for configuration management.
6. *ISO 10011-1:1990,* Guidelines for auditing quality systems — Part 1: Auditing''[1].
7. *ISO 10011-2:1991.* Guidelines for auditing quality systems— Part 2: Qualification criteria for quality systems auditors^.
8. *ISO 10011-3:1991,* Guidelines for auditing quality systems — Part 3: Management of audit programmes''

9. *ISO 10012-1:1992,* Quality assurance requirements for measuring equipment— Part 1: Metrological confirmation system for measuring equipment.
10. *13010012-2:1997,* Quality assurance for measuring equipment— Part 2- Guidelines 'or control of measurement processes.
11. *ISO 10013:1995,* Guidelines for developing quality manuals.
12. *SO/TR 10014:1998.* Guidelines for managing the economics of quality.
13. *ISO 10015:1999.* Quality management — Guidelines for training.
14. *ISO/TR 10017:1999.* Guidance on statistical-techniques for ISO 9001:1994.
15. *ISO 14001:1996,* Environmental management systems — Specification with guidance for use.
16. *I F-C G0300-1 :—*[2]. Dep.. ndabillty management — Part 1: Dependability programme management.
17. Quality Management Principles Brochure.
18. ***ISO 9000 + ISO 14000 News* (a bimonthly publication which provides comprehensive coverage of international developments relating to ISO's management system standards, including news of their implementation by diverse organizations around the world)[4].**
19. **Reference websites : hrtp://.www.iso-ch**

    http://wwwbsi.org uk/iso-lc176-sc2

1. *To ho revised as ISO 19011.* Guidelines on quality anchor environmental management systems auditing.
2. *To be published. (Revision of ISO 9000-4:1993)*
3. *Available from website http://www.iso.ch*
4. *Available from ISO Central Secretariat (sales@iso.ch).*

General

Commission of the European Communities

Committee for Proprietary Medicinal Preparations (CPMP). 4. Analytical validation. Note for guidance. In : The rules governing medicinal products in the European Community. Brussels, CEC (III/844/87-EN, Final, August 1989; Addendum, July 1990).

Committee for proprietary Medicinal Preparations (CPMP). 5. Investigation of bioavailability and bioequivalence. Note for guidance. In: The rules governing medicinal products in the European Community. Brussels, CEC (revised 1991; Volume ill, Addendum No.2, 1992).

Germany

Betriebsverordnung für pharmazeutische Unternehmer. [Factory regulations for pharmaceutical manufacturers] Bonn, §5 and §6, Ministry of Health, 1985, and amendments (in German).

- Basic text : March 9, 1985. Bundesgesetzblatt, 1985,1:546.
- First amendment : March 25, 1988. Bundesgesetzblatt, 1988,1:840.
- Reunification Treaty : August 31, 1990. Bundesgesetz:blatt, 1990,11:885, 1084.
- Second amendment : July 13, 1994. Bundesgesetz:blatt, 1994,1:1560.
- German Pharmaceutical Law, 5th amendment, M. 4, No.1, August 9, 1994. Bundesgesetzblatt, 1994,1:2071.

International Pharmaceutical Federation

Didiog N et al. Komitee für Laboratorien und Offizielle Medikamenten- kontrondienste und der Sektion der Industrieapotheker der FIP. Guidelines for Good Validation Practice (GVP). In: Feiden K.Validation, FIP experience and application in the *FR Germany. Drugs made in Germany.* 1983, **XXVI**:80-85.

Feiden K. Betriebsverordnung für pharmazeutische Unternehmer, Rechtsvorschriften mit speziellen Begrlindungen, erganzenden internationalen Richdinien und einer Einfuhrung. [Factory Regulations for Pharmaceutical Manufacturers, legal provisions with special explanations, complementary international guidelines and an introduction.) In : *PIC- Richtlinien fUr die gute Validierungspraxis. [PIC guidelines on good validation practice],* 3rd ed. Stuttgart, Deutscher ApothekerVerlag, 1991:109-112 (in German).

Richtlinien fur die gute Validierungs-Praxis. [Guidelines on good validation practice.) Pharmazeutische Industrie, 1980, 42(10):982-984 (in German).

Nigeria

Good manufacturing practice for Nigerian pharmaceutical manufacturers. Lagos, Manufacturers' Association of Nigeria, 1991.

Pharmaceutical Inspection Convention

Validation. The collected papers given at a seminar held in Dublin from 14 to 17 June 1982. Geneva, PIC.

Sweden

Validation and qualification processes. Stockholm, Association of Swedish Pharmaceutical Industry [Läkemedelindustriföreningen), 1986.

United States Food and Drug Administration

General principles of validation. Rockville, MD, Center for Drug Evaluation and Research (CDER),1987.

Validation of process and control procedures. Rockville, MD, CDER, 1994.

Guide to inspeaions of bulk pharmaceutical chemicals. Rockville, MD, CDER, 1994.

USSR (former)

Good manufacturing practices. Normative document. Moscow, Ministry of Medical Industry, 1991 (PD 64-125-91, in Russian).

World Health Organization

Good manufacturing practices for pharmaceutical products. In : *WHO Expert Committee on SpecIfications for Pharmaceutical Preparations. Thirty-second report.* Geneva, World Health Organization, 1992: 14-79 (WHO Technical Report Series, No. 823).

Miscellaneous

Barr DB, Crabbs WC, Cooper C. FDA regulation of bulk pharmaceutical chemical production. Pharmaceutical technology, 1993, **17**(9):57-70.

Berry IR, Nash RA, eds. Pharmaceutical process validation, 2nd ed. New York, Marcel Dekker, 1993.

Broker CG. Validation in perspective. Journal of parenteral science and technology, 1981, **35**(4):167-169.

Khan MSP. *Assurance of qua'lity pharmaceuticals. Total quality approach.* Chittagong, Bangladesh, Signet Press, 1990.

Martinez ER. An FDA perspective on bulk pharmaceutical chemical <lMPs, control and validation. *Pharmaceutical engineering*, 1994, **14**(5/6):8-14.

Maynard DW. Validation master planning. *Journal of parenteral science and technology*, 1993,47(2):84-88.

Sucker H. *Praxis der Validierung. [Val,dauon in pracuce.]* Stuttgart, Wissenschaftliche Verlagsgesellschaft, 1983 (in German).

Process Validation

Commission of the European Communities

Committee for Proprietary Medicinal Preparations (CPMP). Development pharmaceutics and process validation. Guidelines on the quality, safety and efficacy of medicinal products for human use. In : *The rules governing medicinal products in the European Community,* Vol. III. Brussels, CEC,1989,

Germany

Arbeitsausschuss Phytopharmaka des Bundesverbandes der Pharmazeutischen Industrie. *Leitlinlt-n zur Herste/lung und Analytik van Phytopharmaka. [Guidelines on the manufacture and analysis of phytopharmaceutics.] Pharmazeutische Industrie,* 1989, **51**(7): 731-734 (in German).

Pharmaceutical Manufacturers Association, USA

Concepts for the process validation of bulk phannaceutical chemicals. Washington, DC, Pharmaceutical Research and Manufacturers of America, 1993 (December):34-40.

United States Food and Drug Administration

Guidelines on general principles of process validation. Rockville, MD, Center for Drug Evaluation and Research, 1987.

Miscellaneous

Akers J, McEntire J, Sorer G. Biotechnology product validation. Part I. Identifying the pitfalls. *Phannaceutical technology Europe*, 1994, 6(2):32-34.

Berry I. Validation : practical applications to pharmaceutical products. *Drug development and industrial pharmacy*, 1988,14(2&3):377-389.

Bias-Imhoff U, Glanzmann G, Woiwode W. Annual product review. *Phannazeutische Industrie*, 1992, 54(2): 177-182.

Chapman KG. The PAR approach to process validation. *Pharmaceutical technology*, 1984, 8(12):22-36.

Chiu YH. Validation of the fermentation process for the production of recombinant DNA drugs. *Phannaceutical technology*, 1988,12(6):132-138.

Cipriano PA. Process validation begins with initial plant design. Phannaceutical engineerzng,1982,.2(3):2.

Loftus BT. Process validation. *Phannazeutische Industrie*, 1980, 42(11a):1202-1205.

Melliger GW. Process validation-practical experience in industry. Phannazeutische Industrie, 1980, 42(l1a): 1199-1202.

Morris JM. Development pharmaceutics and process validation. Drug development ana' zndustnal phannacy, 1990, 16(11):1749-1750.

Sharp JR. *The problems of process validation.* The pharmaceutical joumal, 1986, 1:43-45.

Validation of Non-sterile Processes

Feiden K. Validierung als Beitrag zur Arzneimittel-Sicherheit. [Validation as a contribution to the safety of medicines.] In: *Qualifizzerung und Valzdierung bei der Herstellung jliJssiger und halbfester Arzneifonnen. [Qualification and validation in the manufacturing of liquid and semiliquid finished dosage fonns.]* Heidelberg, Concept, 1987 (in German).

Simmons PL. Solid process validation. *Pharmaceutical engineenng*, 1981, 1(4):38-39, 41.

Thieme H. Implementation of a validation of equipment demonstrated on a Diosna P 600. *Pharmazeutische Industrie,* 1982,44(9):919-924 (in German).

Validation of Sterile Processes

International Pharmaceutical Federation

FIP Committee on Microbial Purity. Validation and environmental monitoring of aseptic processes *Journal of parenteral science and technology*, 1990, 44(5):272-277; *Pharmazeutische Industrie,* 1990, 52(8):1001-1005 (in German); Pharmaceutica acta helvetica, 1990,65(12):327-333 (in French).

United States Food and Drug Administration

Center for Drug Evaluation and Research (CDER). Guideline for submitting documentation for sterilization process validation in application for human and veterinary drug products. *Federal register,* 1993,58(231, December 3):63996-64002.

FDA-Rtchtlinie /iir miltets aseptischer Verfahren hergestellte Arzneimittel. [FDA guideline on stenle drug products produced by aseptic processing.] Pharmazeutische Industrie, 1987, 49(12):1237-1246. (in German).

Guideline on sterile drug products produced by aseptic processing. Rockville, MD, CDER, 1987.

Stenlization process validation. Recommendations for information to be submitted to human and vetennary drug appllcations. Rockville, MD, Center for Veterinary Medicine, CDER, 1993.

World Health Organization

Sterile pharmaceutical products [Section 17 of Good manufacturing practices for pharmaceutical products]. In : *WHO Expert Committee on Specifications for Pharmaceutical Preparations.* Thirty-second report. Geneva, World Health Organization, 1992:59-72. (WHO Technical Report Series, No. 823).

Miscellaneous

Agalloco JP, Akers J. Current practices in the validation of aseptic processes--1992. *Journal of parenteral science and technology,* 1993, 47:51-S21.

Carleton FJ, Agalloco JP. *Validation of aseptic pharmaceutical processes.* New York, Marcel Dekker. 1986,

Carleton FJ et al. *Design concepts for the validation of a water for injectlon system.* Philadelphia, Parenteral Drug Association, 1983 (Technical Report No.4).

Gail L, Wallhiusser KII, Klavehn M. Die Validierung von Trockenhitze-Sterilisatoren. [The validation of dry-heat sterilizers.] *Pharmazeuttsche Industrie,* 1982, 44:613-618 (in German).

Lingnau J. Standard versus non-standard sterilization processes. *Pharmazeutische Industrie,* 1991,53(8):771-775.

Seyfarth H. Validation of aseptic filling for sterile drugs. Part 1. Sterile media fill. *Pharmazeutische Industrie,* 1987,49(11):1176-1183 (in German).

Seyfarth H. Validation of aseptic filling for sterile drugs. Part 2. Environment monitoring. *Pharmazeutische Industrie*, 1988, 50(7): 851-.,863 (in Genran).

Simmons PL. The secret of successful sterilizer validation. *Pharmaceutical engineering*, 1980, 1(1):1,

Tetzlaff RF. Regulatory aspects of aseptic processing. *Pharmaceutical technology*, 1984, 8(11):38-44

Wallhäusser KH. Validation procedure for control of sterilization by filtration. *Pharmazeutzsche Industrie,* 1982,44(4):401-404 (in German).

Validation of Cleaning Processes

Sweden

Valtdation of cleaning methods for process equipment in pharmaceutical manufactunng, Stockholm, Association of Swedish Pharmaceutical Industry [Lakemedel-industriföreningen], 1991,

United States Food and Drug Administration

Guide to inspections of valldation of cleaning processes. Rockvi1le, MD, Division of Field Investigation, 1993.

Miscellaneous

Adner N, Sofer G. Biotechnology product validation. Part 3: chromatography cleaning validation. *Pharmaceutical technology Europe,* 1994, 6(4):22-28.

Baseman HJ. SIP/CIP validation.[1] *Pharmaceutical engineering*, 1992, 12(2):37-46.

Fourman GL, Mullen MV. Determining cleaning validation acceptance limits for pharmaceutical manufacturing operations. Pharmaceutical technology, 1993, 17(4):54-60.

LeBlanc DA, Danforth DD, Smith JM. Cleaning technology for pharmaceutical manufacturing. *Pharmaceutical technology*, 1993, 17(7):84-91.

McCormick PY, Cullen LF. Cleaning validation. In: Berry IR, Nash RA, eds. *Pharmaceutical process validation*, 2nd ed. New York, Marcel Dekker, 1993:319-349.

Seiberling DA. Alternatives to conventional process/CIP[2] design-for improved cleanability. *Pharmaceutical engineering*, 1992, 12(2):16-26.

---

[1]CIP = Cleaning in place/position ;

SIP = Steritizing/steaming in place/position.

[2]CIP = Cleaning in place/position

Smith JA. A modified swabbing technique for validation of detergent residues in clean-place systems. *Pharmaceutical technology*, 1992, 16(1):60-66.

Zeller AO. Cleaning validation and residue limits. A contribution to current discussions. *Pharmaceutical technology,* 1993, 17(10):70-78; *Pharmaceutical technology international,* 1993,17(11):1S-21.

Validation of Analytical Procedures

World Health Organization

Validation of analytical procedures used in the examination of pharmaceutical materials. In: *WHO Expert Committee on Specifications /or Pharmaceutical Preparations. Thirty-second report*. Geneva, World Health Organization, 1992:117-121 (WHO Technical Report Series, No. 823).

Miscellaneous

Grinun W, Schepky G. Stabilitiitspriifung in der Pharmazie. [Stability testing in pharmacy.]. Aulendorf,Germany, Editio Cantor, 1980:335-348 (in German).

Lachman L et al. Quality control charts. In : *The theory and practice of industnal pharmary*. Philadelphia, Lea & Febiger, 1986:817-824.

Quality control methods. In : *Remington's pharmaceutical science*, 18th ed. Easton, PA, Mack, 1990:128-129.

Seely RJ et al. Validation of chromatography resin useful life. In : Biotechnology product validation, part 7. *Pharmaceutical technology Europe*, 1994,6(11):32-38:

Validation of Computerized Systems and Computer-Assisted Processes

United States Food and Drug Administration

A guide to inspection of software development activities (the software liferycle). Rockville, MD, Center for Drug Evaluation and Research (CDER), 1987.

CDER. Guide to inspection of computerized systems in drug processing. *Pharmaceutical industry,* 1983, 1:39-68.

Computerized drug processing : source code for process control application programs. Compliance Policy Guide No. 7132a.15. *Federal register*, 1987,52(95):18612.

Guidance manual : CANDA, computer assisted new drug applications. Rockville, MD, CDER, 1992:1-103.

Points to consider : computer assisted submissions /or license applications. Rockville, MD, Center for Biologics Evaluation and Research, 1990.

Software development activities, reference materials and training aids for investigators. Rockville, MD, Division of Field Investigations, 1987.

Miscellaneous

Christ GA, Unkehcb H-D, Wolf H. Computer-Validierung. [Computer validation.] *Pharmazeutische Industrie,* 1993,55(7):640-644.

Fry EM. FDA regulation of computer systems in drug manufacturing. *Pharmaceutical engineering.* 1988,8{5):47-50.

Geachwandtner R et al. Validation of computer-assisted production processes in pharmaceutical manufacturing. *Pharmazeutische Industrie,* 1989, .51(8):911-913.

Isaacs A. Validation machinery with electronic control systems. *Manufactunng chemIstry.* 1992, 2:19-27.

Kuzel NR. Fundamentals of computer system validation and documentation in the pharmaceutical industry. *Pharmaceutical technology,* 1985, 9(9):60-76.

Motise Pl. What to expect when FDA audits computer-controlled processes. *Pharmaceutical manufacturing,* 1982, 7(7):33-35.

Passing H, Unkelbach H-D. Software-Validierung aus dem Blickwinkel der GLP- bzw. GMP-Richtlinien. [Software validation from the point of view of GLP or GMP guide-lines.] *Pharmaceutische Industrie,* 1987,49(6):590-595 (in German).

Tetzlaff RF. GMP documentation requirements for automated systems. Part I. *Pharmaceutical technology,* 1992, 16(3):112-124.

Tetzlaff RF. GMP documentation requirements for automated systems. Part II. *Pharmaceutical technology,* 1992, 16(4):60-72; Pharmaceutical technology International, 1992, 16(9):30-38.

Tetzlaff RF. GMP documentation requirements for automated systems. Inspections of computerized laboratory systems. Part III. *Pharmaceutical technology international,* 1992, 16(10):36-50.

References

1. W.A. Shewhart: The economic control at quality of manufactured product D. Van Nostrand company. Inc. New York (1991).
2. Duncan, A.J: Quality control and Industrial statistics. R.D. Irwin Inc., Home wood Illinois (1965).
3. Wermimont, G: Use of control charts in analytical analysis. Industrial and Engineering chemistry analytical edition 18 (1976) : 587-592.
4. ASTM (American Society for Testing Materials) Standard methods for the examination of water and waste water 14th edition (1975) 105 B : 26-33.
5. Woodword, R.H and P.L Goldsmith : Cumulative sum techniques, mathematical and statistical techniques for industry. Monograph No. 3, Oliver and Boyd for ICI Edinburgh (1972).
6. Lucas J.M, : A modified 'V' – mask control scheme, Technometrics, 15 (1973) : 833-847.
7. Juran J.D, F.M. Gryna and R.S Bingham (Herausgeber): Quality control handbook. McGraw -Hill Book Company, New York (1975).
8. Inhorn St. (Editor): Quality assurance practices for health. Laboratories American Public Health Association (1978).

9. Reed A.H and R.J Henry,: Accuracy, Precision, Quality control and miscellaneous Statistics. Clinical Chemistry, Principles and Technics. Chapter 12, 287-341.
10. EPA, US (Environmental protection Agency): Handbook for analytical quality control in water and waste water laboratories. EPA-600/4-79-019. Office of research and development. Cincinnati, Ohio 45268 (1979).
11. Cheesman R.V, A.L. Wilson, Manual on analytical quality control for the water Industry, Water research center technical report. TR 66 Medmenhum (1978).
12. ASTM STP 15D: Manual on presentation of data and control chart analysis. American Society of Testing and Materials (1976).
13. Van Dobben de Bruyn C.S: Cumulative sum Techniques : Theory and practice. Griffins' Statistical monographs and courses No. 24, Charles Griffin, London (1968).
14. Jardine A.K.S, J. D. Mac Farlane, C.S. Greensted, : Statistical methods for quality control. The Pitman Press Bath, U.K (1975).
15. Page E. S : Continuous inspection schemes. Biometrika 41 (1954) 100 –115.
16. Whithehead, T. P, Haeckel, and Woodward : Quality control in clinical chemistry. John Wiley & Sons New York, London, (1977).
17. Bermand G.A. control cleans and statistics process J.R. Statist. SOC. B 21 (1959) 239-27.

Subject Index

C

D

E

F

G

H

I

L

M

N

O

P

Q

R

S

T

U

V

Symbols

9 789352 300730

Printed at Repro India Ltd.